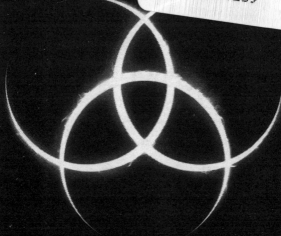

THE STRAIN

JULY

FX

FEARLESS

#TheStrain

Scan code for more info

By Guillermo del Toro and Chuck Hogan

The Night Eternal
The Fall
The Strain

Also by Chuck Hogan

Devils in Exile
The Killing Moon
Prince of Thieves
The Blood Artists
The Standoff

GUILLERMO DEL TORO

CHUCK HOGAN

THE
FALL

Book II of The Strain Trilogy

HARPER

An Imprint of HarperCollinsPublishers

This one is for Lorenza, with all my love.
—GDT
For my four favorite creatures.
—CH

This is a work of fiction. Names, characters, places, and incidents are products of the authors' imagination or are used fictitiously and are not to be construed as real. Any resemblance to actual events, locales, organizations, or persons, living or dead, is entirely coincidental.

HARPER

An Imprint of HarperCollins*Publishers*
195 Broadway
New York, New York 10007

Copyright © 2010 by Guillermo del Toro and Chuck Hogan
ISBN 978-0-06-234462-5

First Harper special premium printing: July 2014
First Harper premium printing: July 2011
First Harper mass market international printing: June 2011
First William Morrow paperback international printing: October 2010
First William Morrow special paperback printing: October 2010
First William Morrow hardcover printing: October 2010

Printed in the United States of America

Visit Harper paperbacks on the World Wide Web at
www.harpercollins.com

10 9 8 7 6 5 4

Extract from the diary of Ephraim Goodweather

Friday, November 26

It took the world just sixty days to end. And we were there to account for it—our omissions, our arrogance . . .

By the time the crisis went to Congress, and was analyzed, legislated, and ultimately vetoed, we had already lost. The night belonged to them.

Leaving us longing for daylight when it was ours no more . . .

All this mere days after our "uncontestable video evidence" reached the world—its truth drowned in thousands of smirking rebuttals and parodies that YouTube'd us beyond all hope.

It became a Late Night pun, smart-asses that we

were, hardy-har-har—until dusk fell upon us and we turned to face an immense, uncaring void.

The first stage of public response to any epidemic is always Denial.

The second, Search For Blame.

All the usual scarecrows were trotted out as distractions: economic woes, social unrest, the racial scapegoating, terrorist threats.

But in the end, it was just us. All of us. We allowed it to happen because we never believed it could happen. We were too smart. Too advanced. Too strong.

And now the darkness is complete.

There are no longer any givens, any absolutes—no root to our existence. The basic tenets of human biology have been rewritten, not in DNA code but in blood and in virus.

Parasites and demons are everywhere. Our future is no longer the natural organic decay of death but a complex and diabolical transmutation. An infestation. A becoming.

They have taken from us our neighbors, our friends, our families. They wear their faces now, the faces of our familiars, our Dear Ones.

We have been turned out of our homes. Cast out of our own kingdom, we roam the outlands in search of a miracle. We survivors are bloodied, we are broken, we are defeated.

But we are not turned. We are not Them.

Not yet.

This is not intended as a record or a chronicle, but as a lamentation, the poetry of fossils, a reminiscence of the end of the era of civilization.

The dinosaurs left behind almost no trace of themselves. A few bones preserved in amber, the contents of their stomachs, their waste.

I only hope that we may leave behind something more than they did.

GRAY SKIES

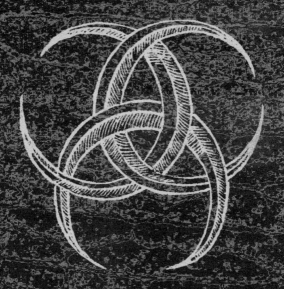

THURSDAY, NOVEMBER 4

*M*irrors are the bearers of bad news, thought Abraham Setrakian, standing under the greenish fluorescent wall lamp, staring into his bathroom mirror. An old man looking into older glass. The edges were blackened with age, a corruption creeping ever closer to the center. To his reflection. To him.

You will die soon.

The silver-backed looking glass showed him that much. Many times he had been close to death, *or worse;* but this was different. In his image he saw this inevitability. And still, somehow, Setrakian found comfort in the truth of the old mirrors. They were honest and pure. This one was a magnificent piece, turn-of-the-century, quite heavy, strung from the wall by corded wire, hanging off the old tile at a downward angle. There were, hung from walls and standing on the floors and leaning against bookshelves, some eighty silver-backed mirrors arranged throughout his living quarters. He collected them compulsively. As people who have walked through a desert know the value of water, so Setrakian found it impossible to pass up the acquisition of a silver looking-glass—especially a smaller, portable one.

But, more than that, he relied upon their most ancient quality.

Contrary to popular myth, vampires certainly do have reflections. In mass-produced, modern mirrors, they appear no different than they do to the eye. But in silver-backed glass, their reflections are distorted. Some physical property of the silver projects these virus-laden atrocities with visual interference—like a warning. Much like the looking glass in the Snow White story, a silver-backed mirror cannot tell a lie.

And so, Setrakian looked at his face in the mirror—between the thick porcelain sink and the counter that held his powders and salves, the rubs for his arthritis, the heated liniment to soothe the pain in his gnarled joints—and studied it.

Here he confronted his fading strength. The acknowledgment that his body was just that: a body. Aged and weakening. Decaying. To the point where he was unsure if he would survive the corporeal trauma of a turning. Not all victims do survive it.

His face. Its deep lines like a fingerprint—the thumb of time stamped firmly onto his visage. He had aged twenty additional years overnight. His eyes appeared small and dry, yellowed like ivory. His pallor was off, and his hair lay against his scalp like fine silver grass matted down by a recent storm.

Pic—pic—pic . . .

He heard death calling. He heard the cane. His heart.

He looked at his twisted hands, molded by sheer will to fit and hold the handle of that silver cane sword—but able to do little else with any dexterity.

The battle with the Master had weakened him greatly. The Master was stronger even than Setrakian had remembered or presumed. He had yet to process his theories spawned by the Master's survival in direct sunlight—sunlight that weakened and marked him, but did not obliterate him. The virus-smashing ultraviolet rays should have cut through him like the power of ten thousand silver swords—and yet the terrible creature had withstood it and escaped.

What is life, in the end, but a series of small victories and larger failures? But what else was there to do? Give up?

Setrakian never gave up.

Second-guessing was all he had at the moment. If only he had done *this* instead of *that.* If he could have somehow dynamited the building once he knew that the Master was inside. If Eph had allowed him to expire rather than saving him at that last critical moment . . .

His heart was racing again, just thinking of lost opportunities. Fluttering and skipping beats. Lurching. Like an impatient child inside him, wanting to run and run.

Pic—pic—pic . . .

A low hum purred above the heartbeat.

Setrakian knew it well: this was the prelude to oblivion, to waking up inside an emergency room, if there were any still operating . . .

With a stiff finger, he fished a white pill out of his box. Nitroglycerin prevented angina by relaxing the vessels carrying blood to his heart, allowing them to dilate, increasing flow and oxygen supply. A sublingual tablet, he placed it underneath his dry tongue, to dissolve.

There was immediately a sweet, tingling sensation. In a few minutes, the murmur in his heart would subside.

The fast-acting nitro pill reassured him. All this second-guessing, this recrimination and mourning: it was a waste of brain activity.

Here he was now. His adopted Manhattan called to him, crumbling from within.

It was a few weeks now since the 777 had touched down at JFK. Since the arrival of the Master and the start of the outbreak. Setrakian had foreseen it from the first news report, as surely as one intuits the death of a loved one when the phone rings at an odd hour. News of the dead plane gripped the city. Just minutes after landing safely, the plane had shut down completely, sitting dark on the taxiway. The Centers for Disease Control and Prevention boarded the plane in contact suits and found all passengers and crew dead, but for four "survivors." These survivors were not well at all, their disease syndrome only augmented by the Master. Hidden inside his coffin within the cargo hold of the airplane, the Master had been delivered across the ocean thanks to the wealth and influence of Eldritch Palmer: a dying man who had chosen not to die but instead to trade human control of the planet for a taste of eternity. After a day's incubation, the virus activated in the dead passengers and they arose from their morgue tables and carried the vampiric plague into the city streets.

The full extent of the plague was known to Setrakian, but the rest of the world resisted the horrible truth. Since then, another airplane had shut down soon after landing at London's Heathrow Airport, stopping dead on the taxiway to the gate. At Orly Airport, an Air France jet arrived stillborn. At Narita International Airport in Tokyo. At Franz Joseph Strauss in Munich. At the famously secure Ben Gurion International in Tel Aviv, where counterterrorist commandos stormed the darkened airliner on the tarmac to find all 126 passengers dead or unresponsive. And yet no alerts were issued to search the cargo areas, or to destroy the airplanes outright. It was happening too fast, and disinformation and disbelief ruled the day.

And on it went. In Madrid. Beijing. Warsaw.

Moscow. Brasília. Auckland. Oslo. Sofia. Stockholm. Reykjavik. Jakarta. New Delhi. Certain more militant and paranoid territories had correctly initiated immediate airport quarantines, cordoning off the dead jets with military force, and yet . . . Setrakian couldn't help but suspect that these landings were as much a tactical distraction as an attempt at infection. Only time would tell if he was correct—though, in truth, there was precious little time.

By now, the original *strigoi*—the first generation of vampires, the Regis Air victims, and their Dear Ones—had begun their second wave of maturation. They were becoming more accustomed to their environment and new bodies. Learning to adapt, to survive—to thrive. They attacked at nightfall, the news reported "rioting" in large sectors of the city, and this was partially true—looting and vandalism ran rampant in broad daylight—but no one pointed out that activity spiked at night.

Because of these disruptions occurring nationwide, the country's infrastructure was beginning to crumble. Food delivery lines were broken, distribution delayed. As absences increased, available manpower suffered and electrical outages and brownouts went unserviced. Police and fire response times were down, and incidences of vigilantism and arson up.

Fires burned. Looters prevailed.

Setrakian stared into his face, wishing he could once again glimpse the younger man within. Perhaps even the boy. He thought of young Zachary Goodweather, just down the hall in the spare bedroom. And, somehow, the old man at the end of his life felt sorry for the boy—eleven years old but already at the end of childhood. Tumbling from grace, stalked by an undead thing occupying the body of his mother . . .

Setrakian stepped out to the dressing area of his bedroom, finding his way to a chair. He sat with one hand covering his face, waiting for the disorienting sensation to pass.

Great tragedy leads to feelings of isolation, which sought to envelop him now. He mourned his long-lost wife, Miriam. Memories of her face had been crowded out of his mind by the few photographs in his possession, which he referred to often and which had the effect of freezing her image in time without ever truly capturing her being. She had been the love of his life. He was a lucky man; it was a struggle sometimes to remember this. He had courted and married a beautiful woman. He had seen beauty and he had seen evil. He had witnessed the best and the worst of the previous century, and he had survived it all. Now he was witnessing the end.

He thought of Ephraim's ex-wife, Kelly, whom Setrakian had met once in life and once again in death. He understood the man's pain. He understood the pain of this world.

Outside, he heard another automobile crash. Gunshots in the distance, alarms ringing insistently—cars, buildings—all going unanswered. The screams that split the night were the last cries of humanity. Looters were taking not only goods and property—they were looting souls. Not taking possessions—but taking possession.

He let his hand fall, landing upon a catalog on the small side table. A Sotheby's catalog. The auction was to be held in just a few days. This was not a coincidence. None of it was coincidence: not the recent occultation, not the conflict overseas, not the economic recession. Like orderly dominoes we fall.

He lifted the auction catalog and searched for a particular page. In it, without any accompanying illustration, was listed an ancient volume:

Occido Lumen (1667)—A compleat account of the first rise of the Strigoi and full confutation of all arguments produced against their existence, translated by the late Rabbi Avigdor Levy. Private collection. Illuminated manuscript, original binding. In view upon appointment. Estimated $15–$25M

This very book—not a facsimile, not a photograph—was crucial to understanding the enemy, the *strigoi*. And vanquishing it.

The book was based on a collection of ancient Mesopotamian clay tablets first discovered in jars inside a cave in the Zagros Mountains in 1508. Written in Sumerian and extremely fragile, the tablets were traded to a wealthy silk merchant, who traveled with them throughout Europe. The merchant was found strangled in his quarters in Florence and his warehouses set on fire. The tablets, however, survived in the possession of two necromancers, the famous John Dee and a more obscure acolyte known to history as John Silence. Dee was Queen Elizabeth I's consultant, and, unable to decipher them, kept the tablets as a magical artifact until 1608 when, forced by poverty, he sold them—through his daughter Katherine—to the learned Rabbi Avigdor Levy in the old ghetto of Metz, in Lorraine, France. For decades, the rabbi meticulously deciphered the tablets, utilizing his unique abilities—it would be almost three centuries before others could finally be able to decipher similar tablets—and eventually presented his findings in manuscript form as a gift for King Louis XIV.

Upon receipt of the text, the king ordered the elderly rabbi's imprisonment and the destruction of the tablets, as well as of the rabbi's entire library of texts and devotional artifacts. The tablets were pulverized, and the manuscript languished in a vault alongside many forbidden treasures. Secretly, Mme de Montespan, the king's mistress and an avid dabbler in the occult, orchestrated the retrieval of the manuscript in 1671. It remained in the hands of La Voisin, a midwife who was de Montespan's sorceress and confidante, until her exile following her implication in the hysteria surrounding the Affaire des Poisons.

The book subsequently resurfaced briefly in 1823, appearing in the possession of the notorious London reprobate and scholar William Beckford. It appeared listed as part of the library in Fonthill Abbey, Beckford's palace of excess, where he accumulated natural and unnatural curiosities, forbidden books, and shocking objets d'art.

The Gothic Revival construction and its contents were sold to an arms dealer in order to satisfy a debt, and the book remained lost for nearly a century. It was listed erroneously, or perhaps surreptitiously, under the title *Casus Lumen* as part of a 1911 auction in Marseille, but the text was never produced for display and the auction summarily canceled after a mysterious outbreak gripped the city. In the ensuing years, the manuscript was widely believed to have been destroyed. Now it was at hand, right here, in New York.

But $15 million? $25 million? Impossible to get. There had to be some other way . . .

His greatest fear, which he dared share with no one, was that the battle, begun so long ago, was already lost. That this was all an endgame, that humanity's king was already in check, yet stubbornly playing out its few remaining moves upon the global chessboard.

Setrakian closed his eyes against a humming in his ears. But the humming persisted—in fact, grew stronger.

The pill had never had this effect on him before.

Once he realized this, Setrakian stiffened and rose to his feet.

It was not the pill at all. The hum was all around him. Low-grade, but there.

They were not alone.

The boy, thought Setrakian. With great effort, he pushed himself up and out of the chair, starting for Zack's room.

Pic—pic—pic . . .

The mother was coming for her boy.

* * *

Zack Goodweather sat cross-legged in the corner of the roof of the pawnshop building. His dad's computer was open in his lap. This was the only spot in the entire building where he could get connected to the Internet, trespassing on the unsecured home network of a neighbor somewhere on the block. The wireless signal was weak, varying between one and two bars, slowing his Internet search to a crawl.

Zack had been forbidden to use his dad's computer. In fact, he was supposed to be asleep right now. The eleven-year-old had enough difficulty sleeping on normal nights, a decent case of insomnia he'd been hiding from his parents for some time.

Insomni-Zack! The first superhero he ever created. An eight-page color comic written, illustrated, lettered, and inked by Zachary Goodweather. About a teen who patrolled the streets of New York by night, foiling terrorists and polluters. And terrorist polluters. He never could get the blanket cape folds to come out right, but he was passable with faces, and okay with musculature.

This city needed an *Insomni-Zack* now. Sleep was a luxury. A luxury no one could afford—if everyone knew what he knew.

If everyone had seen what he had seen.

Zack was supposed to be sacked out in a goose-down sleeping bag inside a spare bedroom on the third floor. The room smelled like a closet, like an old cedar room in his grandparents' house—one that no one opened anymore except for kids who liked to snoop. The small, oddly angled room had been used by Mr. Setrakian (or Professor Setrakian—Zack still wasn't clear on that part, seeing how the old man ran the first-floor pawnshop) for storage. Tilting stacks of books, many old mirrors, a wardrobe of old clothes, and some locked trunks—really locked, not the fake kind of lock that can be picked with a paper clip and a ballpoint pen (Zack had already tried).

The exterminator, Fet—or V, as he had told Zack to call him—had hooked up an ancient, cartridge-fed, 8-bit Nintendo system to a pawned Sanyo television set with big knobs and dials on the front instead of buttons, all brought up from the showroom downstairs. They expected him to stay put and play *The Legend of Zelda*. But the bedroom door had no lock. His dad and Fet had mounted iron bars onto the wall over the window—mounted them on the inside, rather than the outside, bolted to the wall beams—a cage that Mr. Setrakian said was left over from the 1970s.

They weren't trying to lock him in, Zack knew. They were trying to lock *her* out.

He searched for his dad's professional page at the Centers for Disease Control and Prevention, and got a "Page Not Found." So they had already scrubbed him from the government Web site. News hits for "Dr. Ephraim Goodweather" claimed he was a discredited CDC official who fabricated a video purporting to show a human-turned-vampire being destroyed. It said that he had uploaded it (actually, Zack uploaded the video for him, one that his dad wouldn't let him view) onto the Internet in an attempt to exploit the eclipse hysteria for his own purposes. Obviously, that last part was BS. What "purposes" did his dad have other than trying to save lives? One news site described Goodweather as "an admitted alcoholic involved in a contentious custody battle, who is now believed to be on the run with his kidnapped son." That left Zack with a lump of ice in his chest. The same article went on to say that both Goodweather's ex-wife and her boyfriend were currently missing and presumed dead.

Everything made Zack feel nauseous these days, but the dishonesty of this article was especially toxic to him. All wrong, every last word. Did they really not know the truth? Or . . . did they not care? Maybe they were trying to exploit his parents' trouble *for their own purposes*?

And the talkback? The comments were even worse. He could not deal with the things they were saying about his dad, the righteous arrogance of all these anonymous posters. He had to deal right now with the awful truth about his mom—and the banality of the venom spewed in blogs and forums missed the point completely.

How do you mourn someone who isn't really gone? How do you fear someone whose desire for you is eternal?

If the world knew the truth the way Zack knew the truth, then his dad's reputation would be restored, and his voice heard—but still nothing else would change. His mom, his life, would never be the same.

So, mostly, Zack wanted it all to pass. He wanted something fantastic to happen to make everything right and normal again. As when he was a child—like five or something, he broke a mirror and just covered it with a sheet, then prayed with all his might for its restoration before his parents found out. Or the way he used to wish his parents would fall back in love again. That they would wake up one day and realize what a mistake they had made.

Now he secretly hoped that his dad could do something incredible. Despite everything, Zack still assumed that there was some happy ending awaiting them. Awaiting all of them. Maybe even something to bring Mom back to the way she was.

He felt tears coming, and this time he didn't fight them. He was up on the roof; he was alone. He wanted so badly to see his mother again. The thought terrified him—and yet he yearned for her to come. To look into her eyes. To hear her voice. He wished for her to explain this to him the way she did every troubling thing. *Everything is going to be just fine . . .*

A scream somewhere deep in the night brought him back to the present. He peered uptown, seeing flames on the west side, a column of dark smoke. He looked up. No stars tonight. And only a few airplanes. He had heard fighter jets zooming overhead that afternoon.

Zack rubbed his face in the crook of his elbow sleeve and turned back to the computer. With some quick desktop searching, Zack discovered the folder containing the video file he was not supposed to view. He opened it and heard Dad's voice, and realized Dad was operating the camera. Zack's camera, the one his dad had borrowed.

The subject was hard to see at first, something in the dark inside a shed. A thing leaning forward on its haunches. A guttural growl and a back-of-the-throat hiss. The slinking noise of a chain. The camera zoomed in closer, the dark pixilation improving, and Zack saw its open mouth. A mouth that opened wider than it should, with something resembling a thin silver fish flopping inside.

The shed-thing's eyes were wide and glaring. He mistook their expression for one of sadness at first, and hurt. A collar—apparently, a dog collar—restrained it at the neck, chained to the dirt floor behind it. The creature looked pale inside the dark shed, so bloodless it was nearly glowing. Then came a strange pumping sound— *snap-chunk, snap-chunk, snap-chunk*—and three silver nails, propelled from behind the camera (from Dad?) struck the shed-thing like needle-bullets. The camera view jerked up as the thing roared hoarsely, a sick animal consumed with pain.

"Enough," said a voice on the clip. The voice belonged to Mr. Setrakian, but it was not a tone like anything Zack had ever heard out of the kindly, old pawnbroker's mouth. *"Let us remain merciful."*

Then the old man stepped into view, intoning some words in a foreign, ancient-sounding language—almost like summoning a power or declaring a curse. He raised a silver sword—long and bright with moonlight—and the shed-thing howled as Mr. Setrakian swung the sword with great force . . .

Voices pulled Zack out of the video. Voices from the street below. He shut the laptop and stood, staying back, peering over the raised edge of the roof down to 118th Street.

A group of five men walked up the block toward the pawnshop, trailed by a slow-moving SUV. They carried weapons—guns—and were pounding on every door. The SUV stopped before the intersection, right outside the front of the pawnshop. The men on foot approached the building, rattling the security gates. Calling, "Open up!"

Zack backed away. He turned to go to the roof door, figuring he'd better get back to his room in case anyone came looking.

Then he saw her. A girl, a teenager, high school probably. Standing on the next roof over, across an empty lot around the corner from the shop entrance. The breeze lifted her long nightshirt, ruffling it around her knees, but did not move her hair, which hung straight and heavy.

She stood on the raised edge of the roof. The very edge, balanced perfectly, no wavering in her posture. Poised at the brink, as though wanting to try to make the jump. The impossible leap. Wanting to and knowing she would fail.

Zack stared. He didn't know. He wasn't sure. But he suspected.

He raised a hand anyway. He waved to her.

She stared back at him.

*   *   *

Dr. Nora Martinez, late of the Centers for Disease Control ánd Prevention, unlocked the front door. Five men in combat gear with armored vests and assault weapons stared her down through the security grate. Two of them wore kerchiefs, covering their lower faces.

"Everything all right in there, ma'am?" one of them asked.

"Yes," said Nora, looking for badges or any kind of insignia and seeing none. "So long as this grate holds up, everything is fine."

"We're going door-to-door," said another. "Clearing blocks. Some trouble down that way"—he pointed toward 117th Street—"but we think the worst of it is moving downtown from this direction." Meaning Harlem.

"And you are . . . ?"

"Concerned citizens, ma'am. You don't want to be in here all alone."

"She's not," said Vasiliy Fet, the New York City Bureau of Pest Control Services worker and independent exterminator, appearing behind her.

The men sized up the big man. "You the pawnbroker?"

"My father," said Fet. "What sort of trouble are you seeing?"

"Trying to get a handle on these freaks rioting in the city. Agitators and opportunists. Taking advantage of a bad situation, making it worse."

"You sound like cops," said Fet.

"If you're thinking about leaving town," said

another one, avoiding the topic, "you should go now. Bridges are stacked up, tunnels jammed. Place is going to shit."

Another said, "You should think about getting out here and helping us. Do something about this."

Fet said, "I'll think about it."

"Let's go!" called the driver of the SUV idling in the street.

"Good luck," said one of the men, with a scowl. "You'll need it."

Nora watched them go, then locked the door. She stepped back into the shadows. "They're gone," she said.

Ephraim Goodweather, who had been watching from the side, emerged. "Fools," he said.

"Cops," said Fet, watching them round the street corner.

"How do you know?" asked Nora.

"You can always tell."

"Good thing you stayed out of sight," Nora said to Eph.

Eph nodded. "Why no badges?"

Fet said, "Probably got off shift and huddled up at happy hour, decided this wasn't how they were going to let their city go out. Wives all packed up for Jersey, they've got nothing to do now but bang some heads. Cops feel they run the place. And they're not half wrong. Street-gang mentality. It's their turf and they'll fight for it."

"When you think about it," said Eph, "they're really not that much different than us right now."

Nora said, "Except that they're carrying lead

when they should be wielding silver." She slipped her hand into Eph's. "I wish we could have warned them."

"Trying to warn people is how I got to be a fugitive in the first place," said Eph.

Eph and Nora were the first to board the dead plane after SWAT team members discovered the apparently dead passengers. The realization that the bodies weren't decomposing naturally, coupled with the disappearance of the coffin-like cabinet during the solar occultation, had helped convince Eph that they were facing an epidemiological crisis which could not be explained by normal medical and scientific means. The grudging realization opened him up to the revelations of the pawnbroker, Setrakian, and the terrible truth behind the plague. His desperation to warn the world of the true nature of the disease—the vampiric virus moving insidiously through the city and out into the boroughs—led to a break with the CDC, which then tried to silence him with a trumped-up charge of murder. He had been a fugitive ever since.

He looked to Fet. "Car packed?"

"Ready to go."

Eph squeezed Nora's hand. She did not want to let him go.

Setrakian's voice came down the spiral stairs in back of the showroom. "Vasiliy? Ephraim! Nora!"

"Down here, professor," replied Nora.

"Someone approaches," he said.

"No, we just got rid of them. Vigilantes. Well-armed ones."

"I don't mean someone human," said Setra-kian. "And I cannot find young Zack."

Zack's bedroom door banged open, and he turned. His dad blew in, looking like he expected a fight. "Jeez, Dad," said Zack, sitting up in his sleeping bag.

Eph looked all around the room. "Setrakian said he just looked in here for you."

"Uhh . . ." Zack made a show of rubbing his eye. "Must not have seen me on the floor."

"Yeah. Maybe." Eph looked at Zack a bit longer, not believing him, but clearly with something more pressing on his mind than catching his son in a lie. He walked around the room, checking the barred window. Zack noticed that he held one hand behind his back, and moved in such a way that Zack could not see what he held there.

Nora rushed in behind him, then stopped when she saw Zack.

"What is it?" asked Zack, getting to his feet.

His dad shook his head reassuringly, but the smile came too quickly—just a smile, no levity in his eyes, none at all. "Just looking around. You wait here, 'kay? I'll be back."

He exited, turning in such a way that the thing behind his back remained obscured. Zack wondered: was it the *snap-chunk* thing, or some silver sword?

"Stay put," said Nora, and closed the door.

Zack wondered what it was they were looking for. Zack had heard his mother mention Nora's name once in a fight with his dad—well, not a fight really, since they were already split up, but more of a venting. And Zack had seen his dad kiss her that one time—right before he left them and went off with Mr. Setrakian and Fet. Then she had been so tense and preoccupied the whole time they were gone. And once they returned—everything had changed. Zack's dad had looked so down—Zack never wanted to see him look that way again. And Mr. Setrakian came back sick. Zack, in his subsequent snooping, had caught some of the talk, but not enough.

Something about a "master."

Something about sunlight and failing to "destroy it."

Something about "the end of the world."

As Zack stood alone in the spare room now, puzzling out all these mysteries swirling around him, he noticed a blur in a few of the mirrors hanging on the wall. A distortion, akin to a visual vibration—something that should have been in focus but instead appeared hazy and indistinct in the glass.

Something at his window.

Zack turned, slowly at first—then all at once.

She was clinging to the exterior of the building somehow. Her body was disjointed and distorted, her eyes red and wide and burning. Her hair was falling out, thin and pale now, her schoolteacher dress torn away at one shoulder, her exposed flesh smeared with dirt. The muscles of her neck were swollen and deformed, and blood worms slithered beneath her cheeks, across her forehead.

Mom.

She had come. As he knew she would.

Instinctively, he took a step toward her. Then he read her expression, which all at once transformed from pain into a darkness that could only be described as demonic.

She had noticed the bars.

In an instant, her jaw dropped open—way open, just like in the video—a stinger shooting out from deep beneath where her tongue was. It pierced the window glass with a crack and a tinkle, and kept coming through the hole it punched. Six feet in length, the stinger tapering to a point and snapping at full extension mere inches from his throat.

Zack froze, his asthmatic lungs locked, unable to draw any breath.

At the end of the fleshy shoot, a complicated, double-pronged tip quivered, rooting in the air. Zack remained riveted to the spot. The stinger relaxed and, with a casual, upward nod of her head, she retracted it quickly back into her mouth. Kelly Goodweather thrust her head through the window, crashing out the rest of the glass. She squeezed up inside the open window frame, needing only a few more inches to reach Zack's throat and claim her Dear One for the Master.

Zack was transfixed by her eyes. Red with black points in the center. He searched, vertiginously, for some semblance of *Mom*.

Was she dead, as Dad said? Or alive?

Was she gone forever? Or was she here—right here in the room with him?

GUILLERMO DEL TORO AND CHUCK HOGAN

Was she still his? Or was she now someone else's?

She jammed her head between the iron bars, grinding flesh and cracking bone, like a snake forcing itself into a rabbit's hole, trying desperately to bridge the extra distance between her stinger and the boy's flesh. Her jaw fell again, her glowing eyes settling on the boy's throat, just above his Adam's apple.

Eph came racing back into the bedroom. He found Zack standing there, staring dumbly at Kelly, the vampire squeezing its head between the iron bars, about to strike. Eph pulled a silver-bladed sword from behind his back, yelling, "NO!" and jumping in front of Zack.

Nora burst into the room behind Eph, turning on a Luma lamp, its harsh UVC light humming. The sight of Kelly Goodweather—this corrupted human being, this monster-mother—repulsed Nora, but she advanced, the virus-killing light in her outstretched hand.

Eph, too, moved toward Kelly and her hideous stinger. The vampire went deep-eyed with animal rage.

"OUT! GO BACK!" Eph bellowed at Kelly the way he might at some wild animal trying to enter his house, scavenging for food. He leveled the sword at her and made a run for the window.

With one last, painfully ravenous look at her son, Kelly pulled back from the window cage, just out of Eph's blade's reach—and darted away along the side of the exterior wall.

Nora placed the lamp inside the cage, resting it

upon two intersecting bars so that its killing light filled the space of the smashed window, to keep Kelly from returning.

Eph ran back to his son. Zack's gaze had fallen, his hands at his throat, chest bucking. Eph thought at first it was despair, then realized it was more than that.

A panic attack. The boy was all locked up inside. He was unable to breathe.

Eph looked around frantically, discovering Zack's inhaler on top of the old television. He pressed the device into Zack's hands and guided it to his mouth.

Eph squeezed, and Zack huffed, and the aerosol opened up his lungs. Zack's pallor improved immediately, his airway expanding like a balloon—and Zack slumped, weakened.

Eph set down his sword, steadying the boy—but the revived Zack shoved him away, rushing toward the empty window. "Mom!" he croaked.

Kelly retreated up the brick face of the building, the talons developing out of her middle fingers aiding her ascent as she climbed flat against the building side, like a spider. Fury at the interloper carried her along. She felt—with the intensity of a mother dreaming of a distressed child calling out her name—the exquisite nearness of her Dear One. The psychic beacon that was his human grief. The force of his need for his mother redoubled her unconditional vampiric need for him.

What she saw when she had laid eyes upon Zachary Goodweather again was not a boy. Was not her son, her love. She saw instead a piece of her that stubbornly remained human. She saw something that remained hers by biology, a part of her being forever. Her own blood, only still human-red, not vampire-white. Still carrying oxygen, not food. She saw an incomplete part of her, held back by force.

And she wanted it. She wanted it like crazy.

This was not human love, but vampire need. Vampire longing. Human reproduction spreads outward, creating and growing, while vampiric reproduction operates in the reverse, turning back upon the bloodline, inhabiting living cells and converting them to its own ends.

The positive attractor, love, becomes its opposite, which is not, in fact, hate—nor death. The negative attractor is infection. Instead of sharing love and the joining of seed and egg and the commingling gene pools in the creation of a new and unique being, it is a corruption of the reproductive process. An inert substance invading a viable cell and producing hundreds of millions of identical copies. It is not shared and creative, but violent, destructive. It is a defilement and a perversion. It is biological rape and supplantation.

She needed Zack. As long as he remained unfinished, she remained incomplete.

The Kelly-thing stood poised on the edge of the roof, indifferent to the suffering city all around her. She knew only thirst. A craving, for blood and for her blood kind. This was the frenzy that compelled her; a virus knows only one thing: that it must infect.

She had begun to search for some other way inside this brick box when, from behind the doorway bulkhead, she heard a pair of old shoes crunching gravel.

In the darkness, she saw him well. The old hunter Setrakian appeared with a silver sword, advancing. He meant to pin her against the edge of the roof and the night.

His heat signature was narrow and dull; an aged human, his blood moved slowly. He appeared small, though all humans appeared small to her now. Small and unformed, creatures grasping at the edge of existence, tripping over their paltry intellect. The butterfly with a death's head on its winged back looks at a furry chrysalis with absolute disdain. An earlier stage of evolution, an outmoded model incapable of hearing the soothing exultation of the Master.

Something in her always went back to Him. Some primitive and yet coordinated form of animal communication. The psyche of the hive.

As the old human advanced toward her with his slaying silver blade glowing brightly in her vision, a response came forth, directly from the Master, relayed through her into the mind of the old avenger.

Abraham.

From the Master, and yet—not of his great voice, as Kelly understood it.

Abraham. Don't.

It came as a woman's intonation. Not Kelly's. No voice she had ever heard.

But Setrakian had. She saw it in his heat signature, the way his heart rate quickened.

I live in her too . . . I live in her . . .

The avenger stopped, a hint of weakness coming into his eyes. The Kelly vampire seized on the moment, her chin falling, her mouth jerking open, feeling the impending thrust of her activated stinger.

But then the hunter raised his weapon and came at her with a cry. She had no choice. The silver blade burned in the night of her eyes.

She turned and ran along the edge, turning down and scuttling low along the wall of the building. From the vacant lot below, she looked back once at the old human, his shrinking heat signature, standing alone, watching her go.

Eph went to Zack, pulling on his arm, keeping him back from the scalding UV light of the lamp inside the window cage.

"Get away!" yelled Zack.

"Buddy," said Eph, trying to calm him down, calm them both down. "Guy. Z. Hey."

"You tried to kill her!"

Eph didn't know what to say, because indeed he had. "She's . . . she's dead already."

"Not to me!"

"You saw her, Z." Eph didn't want to have to

talk about the stinger. "You saw it. She's not your mom anymore. I'm sorry."

"You don't have to kill her!" Zack said, his voice still raw from choking.

"I do," said Eph. "I do."

He went to Zack, trying again for some contact, but the boy pulled away. He went instead to Nora, who was handy as a female substitute, and cried into her shoulder.

Nora looked back at Eph with consolation in her eyes, but Eph wouldn't have it. Fet was at the door behind him.

"Let's go," said Eph, rushing from the room.

The Night Squad

THEY CONTINUED UP the street toward Marcus Garvey Park, the five off-duty cops on foot, and the sergeant in his personal vehicle.

No badges. No cruiser cameras. No after-action reports. No inquiries, no community boards, and no Internal Affairs.

This was about force. About setting things right.

"Communicable mania," the feds termed it. "Plague-related dementia."

What happened to good, old-fashioned "bad guys"? That term gone out of style?

The government was talking about deploying the Staties? The National Guard? The Army?

At least give us blue boys a shot first.

"Hey—what the . . . !"

One of them was holding his arm. A deep cut, right through the sleeve.

Another projectile landed at their feet.

"Fucking throwing rocks now?"

They scanned the rooftops.

"There!"

A huge chunk of decorative stone, a fleur-de-lis, came sailing down at their heads, scattering them. The piece shattered onto the curb, rock smacking their shins.

"In here!"

They ran for the door, busted inside. The first man in charged up the stairs to the second-floor landing. There, a teenage girl in a long nightshirt stood in the middle of the hallway.

"Get outta here, honey!" he yelled, pushing right past her, heading for the next flight of stairs. Someone was on the move up there. The cop didn't have to wait for rules of engagement, or justifiable force. He yelled at him to stop, then opened up on the guy, plugging him four times, putting him down.

He advanced on the rioter, all charged up. A black guy with four good hits in his chest. The cop smiled down the gap in the stairs.

"I got one!"

The black guy sat up. The cop backed away, getting off one more round before the guy sprang on him, clutching him, doing something to his neck.

The cop spun, his assault rifle pressed flat between them, feeling the railing give against his hip.

They fell together, landing hard. Another cop turned and saw the suspect on top of the first cop, biting him on the neck or something. Before firing, he looked up to see where they had fallen from—and saw the nightshirt-wearing teen.

She leaped down at him, knocking him flat, straddling him, and clawing at his face and neck.

A third cop came back down the stairs and saw her—then saw the guy behind her with a stinger coming out of his mouth, throbbing as it drained the first cop.

The third cop fired on the teen, knocking her back. He started to go after the other freak when a hand swept down from behind him, a long, talon-like nail slicing open his neck, spinning him into the creature's arms.

Kelly Goodweather, her rage of hunger and blood-need triggered by the yearning for her son, dragged the cop one-handedly into the nearest apartment, slamming the door so that she could feed deeply and without interruption.

The Master—Part I

THE MAN'S LIMBS twitched for the last time, the faint perfume of his final breath escaping his mouth, the death rattle signaling the end of the repast for the Master. The man's inert, nude body, released by the towering shadow, collapsed next to the other four victims similarly at the feet of Sardu.

All of them exhibited the same concussive

stinger mark in the soft flesh of the inside thigh, right on the femoral artery. The popular image of a vampire drinking from the neck was not incorrect, but powerful vampires favored the femoral artery of the right leg. The pressure and oxygenation were perfect, and the flavor was fuller, almost blunt. The jugular, on the other hand, carried impure, tangy blood. Regardless, the act of feeding had long ago lost its thrill for the Master. Many a time the ancient vampire fed without even looking into its victim's eyes—although the adrenaline surge of fear in the victim added an exotic tingle to the metallic flavor of blood.

For centuries, human pain remained fresh and even invigorating: its various manifestations amused the Master, the cattle's delicate symphony of gasps and screams and exhalations still arousing the creature's interest.

But now, especially when it fed like this, en masse, it sought absolute silence. From within, the Master called upon its primal voice—its original voice—the voice of its true self, shedding all other guests within its body and its will. It emitted its murmur: a pulse, a psycho-sedative rumble from within, mental whiplash, paralyzing nearby prey for the longest time in order that the Master could feed at peace.

But in the end, *The Murmur* was to be used cautiously, for it exposed the Master's true voice. Its true self.

It took a bit of time and effort to quiet all the inhabiting voices and discover its own again. This was dangerous, as these voices served as the Master's cloaking device. The voices—including that of Sardu, the boy hunter whose body the Master inhabited—camouflaged the Master's presence, position, and thoughts before the other Ancient Ones. They cloaked him.

It had used *The Murmur* inside the 777 at arrival, and it wielded the pulse-sound now to gain absolute silence and collect its thoughts. The Master could do it here—hundreds of feet below ground level, in a concrete vault at the center of the semi-abandoned charnel house complex. The Master's chamber resided at the center of a labyrinth of curving corralled areas and service tunnels beneath the steer abattoir above them. Blood and residue had once been collected there, but now, after a thorough cleaning in advance of the Master's residency, the structure resembled most closely a small industrial chapel.

The pulsating slash on the Master's back had started healing almost instantly. He never feared any permanent damage from the wound—he never feared anything—and yet the slash would form into a scar, defacing his body like an affront. The old fool and the humans by his side would regret the day they crossed the Master.

The faintest echo of rage—of deep indignation—rippled through its many voices and its single will. The Master felt vexed, a refreshing and energizing sensation. Indignation was not a feeling it experienced often, and thus the Master allowed—even welcomed—this novel reaction.

Quiet laughter rattled through its injured body.

The Master was way ahead of the game, and all of its various pawns were behaving as expected. Bolivar, the energetic lieutenant in his ranks, was proving quite apt at spreading the thirst, and had even collected a few serfs that could do sun chores for them. Palmer's arrogance grew with each tactical advance, yet he remained fully under the Master's control. The Occultation had marked the time for the plan to be set forth. It had defined the delicate, sacred geometry needed, and now— very soon—the earth would burn . . .

On the floor, one of the morsels groaned, unexpectedly clinging to life. Refreshed and delighted, the Master gazed down upon it. In its mind, the chorus of voices restarted. The Master looked upon the man at his feet, and some pain and fear remained in his gaze—an unanticipated treat.

This time, the Master indulged itself, savoring the tangy dessert. Under the vaulted roof of the Charnel House, the Master lifted the body up, carefully laying its hand over the chest, above the heart of the man, and greedily extinguished the rhythm within.

Ground Zero

THE PLATFORM WAS empty when Eph jumped down onto the tracks, following Fet into the subway tunnel leading alongside the construction bathtub of the Ground Zero project.

He never imagined he would return here, to

this place. After everything they had witnessed and encountered before, he could not imagine a force strong enough to compel him to return to the subterranean labyrinth that was the Master's nest.

But calluses form in as little as one day. Scotch had helped. Scotch helped quite a bit.

He walked over black rocks along the same out-of-service track as before. The rats had not returned. He passed the sump hose abandoned by the sandhogs who had also disappeared.

Fet carried his usual steel rod of rebar. Despite the more appropriate and impactful weapons they carried—ultraviolet lamps, silver swords, a nail gun loaded with brads of pure silver—Fet continued to carry his rat stick, though they both knew there were no longer any rats here. Vampires had infested the rats' subterranean domain.

Fet also liked the nail gun. Pneumatic air-powered nail guns required tubing and water. Electric nail guns lacked punch and trajectory. Neither was truly portable. Fet's powder-actuated gun—a weapon from the old man's arsenal of oddities ancient and modern—operated on a shotgun load of gunpowder. Fifty silver nails per load, fed through the bottom like the magazine of an UZI. Lead bullets put holes in vamps, same as humans—but when your nervous system is gone, physical pain is a nonissue, copper-plated projectiles reduced to blunt instruments. A shotgun had stopping power, but unless you severed the head at the neck, pellet blasts didn't kill either. Silver, introduced in the form of an inch-and-a-half brad, killed viruses. Lead bullets made them angry, but silver nails hurt them at something like a genetic level. And, almost as important, at least to Eph: silver scared them. As did ultraviolet light in the pure, shortwave UVC range. Silver and sunlight were the vampire equivalent of the exterminator's rat stick.

Fet had come to them as a city employee, an exterminator who wanted to know what was driving the rats out from underground. He had already run into a few vampires in his subterranean adventures, and his skill set—a dedicated killer of vermin, and an expert in the workings of the city beneath the city—lent itself perfectly to vampire hunting. He was the one who had first led Eph and Setrakian down here in search of the Master's nest.

The smell of slaughter remained trapped in the underground chamber. The charred stench of roasted vampire—and the lingering ammonia odor of the creatures' excrement.

Eph found himself lagging behind, and picked up his pace, sweeping the tunnel with his flashlight, catching up to Fet.

The exterminator chewed an unlit Toro cigar, which he was used to talking around. "You okay?" he asked.

"I'm great," said Eph. "Couldn't be better."

"He's confused. Man, I was confused at that age, and my mother wasn't . . . you know."

"I know. He needs time. And that's just one of many things I can't give him right now."

"He's a good kid. I don't usually like kids, but I like yours."

Eph nodded, appreciative of the effort Fet was putting forth. "I like him too."

"I worry about the old man."

Eph stepped carefully over the loose stones. "It took a lot out of him."

"Physically, sure. But there's more."

"Failure."

"That, yes. Getting so near, after so many years of chasing these things, only to see the Master withstand and survive the old man's best shot. But something else too. There are things he's not telling us. Or hasn't told us yet. I am sure of it."

Eph remembered the king vampire throwing back its cloak in a gesture of triumph, its lily-white flesh cooking in the daylight as it howled at the sun in defiance—then disappearing over the edge of the rooftop. "He thought sunlight would kill the Master."

Fet chewed his cigar. "The sun did hurt it, at least. Who knows how long that thing would have been able to take the exposure. And you— you cut him. With the silver." Eph had gotten in a half-lucky slash across the Master's back, which the sun's subsequent exposure fused into an instant black scar. "If it can be hurt, I guess it can be destroyed. Right?"

"But—isn't a wounded animal more dangerous?"

"Animals, like people, are motivated by pain and fear. But this thing? Pain and fear are where it lives. It doesn't need any additional motivation."

"To wipe us all out."

"I've been thinking a lot about that. Would he want to wipe out all of mankind? I mean—we're his food. We're his breakfast, lunch, and dinner. He turns everyone into vamps, there goes his entire food supply. Once you kill all the chickens, no more eggs."

Eph was impressed by Fet's reasoning, the logic of an exterminator. "He's got to maintain a balance, right? Turn too many people into vampires, you create too great a demand for human meals. Blood economics."

"Unless there's some other fate in store for us. I only hope the old man has the answers. If he doesn't . . ."

"Then nobody does."

They came up to the dingy tunnel junction. Eph held up his Luma lamp, the UVC rays bringing out the wild stains of vampire waste: their urine and excrement, whose biological matter fluoresced under the low light range. The stains were no longer the garish colors Eph remembered. These stains were fading. This meant that no vampires had revisited the spot recently. Perhaps, through their apparent telepathy, they had been warned away by the deaths of the hundreds of fellow creatures that Eph, Fet, and Setrakian had slain.

Fet used his steel rod to poke at the mound of discarded mobile phones, piled up like a cairn. A desultory monument to human futility—as though vampires had sucked the life out of people, and all that was left were their gadgets.

Fet said, quietly, "I've been thinking about

something he said. He was talking about myths from different cultures and ages revealing similar basic human fears. Universal symbols."

"Archetypes."

"That was the word. Terrors common to all tribes and countries, deep in all humans across the board—diseases and plagues, warfare, greed. His point was, what if these things aren't just superstitions? What if they are directly related? Not separate fears linked by our subconscious— but what if they have actual roots in our past? In other words, what if these aren't common myths? What if they are common truths?"

Eph found it difficult to process theory down in the underbelly of the besieged city. "You're saying that he's saying that maybe we've always known . . . ?"

"Yes—always feared. That this threat—this clan of vampires who subsist on human blood, and whose disease possesses human bodies— existed and was known. But as they went underground, or what-have-you, retreating into the shadows, the truth got massaged into myth. Fact became folklore. But this well of fear runs so deeply, throughout all peoples and all cultures, that it never went away."

Eph nodded, interested but also distracted. Fet could stand back and consider the big picture, while Eph's situation was the opposite of Fet's. His wife—his ex-wife—had been taken, turned. And now she was hell-bent on turning her blood, her Dear One, their son. This plague of demons had affected him on a personal level, and he was finding it difficult to focus on anything else, never mind theorizing on the grand scale of things—though that was, in fact, his training as an epidemiologist. But when something this insidious enters your personal life, all superior thinking goes out the window.

Eph found himself increasingly obsessed with Eldritch Palmer, the head of the Stoneheart Group and one of the three richest men in the world—and the man they had identified as the Master's coconspirator. As the domestic attacks had scaled up, doubling each passing night, the strain spreading exponentially, the news insisted on reducing them to mere "riots." This was akin to calling a revolution an isolated protest. They had to know better, and yet someone—it *had* to be Palmer, a man with a vested interest in misleading the American public and the world at large—was influencing the media and controlling the CDC. Only his Stoneheart Group could finance and enforce such a massive campaign of public misinformation about the occultation. Eph had determined, privately, that if they could not readily destroy the Master, well, they could certainly destroy Palmer, who was not only elderly but notoriously infirm. Any other man would have passed on ten years ago, but Palmer's vast fortune and unlimited resources kept him alive, like an antique vehicle requiring round-the-clock maintenance just to keep it running. Life, the doctor in Eph imagined, had become for Palmer something akin to a fetish: How long could he keep going?

Eph's fury at the Master—for turning Kelly, for upending everything Eph believed about science and medicine—was justified but impotent, like shaking his fists at death itself. But condemning Palmer, the Master's human collaborator and enabler, gave Eph's torment a direction and a purpose. Even better, it legitimized a desire for personal revenge.

This old man had shattered Eph's son's life and broken the boy's heart.

They reached the long chamber that was their destination. Fet readied his nail gun and Eph brandished his sword before turning the corner.

At the far end of the low chamber stood the mound of dirt and refuse. The filthy altar upon which the coffin—the intricately carved cabinet had traversed the Atlantic inside the cold underbelly of Regis Air Flight 753, inside which the Master lay buried in cold, soft loam—had lain.

The coffin was gone. Disappeared again, as it had from the secure hangar at LaGuardia Airport. The flattened top of the dirt altar still bore its impression.

Someone—or, more likely, some *thing*—had returned to claim it before Eph and Fet could destroy the Master's resting place.

"He's been back here," said Fet, looking all around.

Eph was bitterly disappointed. He had longed to demolish the heavy cabinet—to turn his wrath on some physical form of destruction, and to disrupt the monster's habitat in some certain way. To let it know that they had not given up, and would never back down.

"Over here," said Fet. "Look at this."

A splashed-out swirl of colors at the base of the side wall, given life by the rays of Fet's lamp wand, indicated a fresh spray of vampire urine. Then Fet illuminated the entire wall with a normal flashlight.

A graffiti mural of wild designs, random in arrangement, covered the stone expanse. Closer, Eph discerned that the vast majority of the figures were variations on a six-pointed motif, ranging from rudimentary to abstract to simply bewildering. Here was something starlike in appearance; there a more amoeba-like pattern. The graffiti spread out across the wide wall in the manner of a thing replicating itself, filling the stone face from bottom to top. Up close, the paint smelled fresh.

"This," said Fet, stepping back to take it all in, "is new."

Eph moved in to examine a glyph at the center of one of the more elaborate stars. It appeared to be a hook, or a claw, or . . .

"A crescent moon." Eph moved his black-light lamp across the complex motif. Invisible to the naked eye, two identical shapes were hidden in the vectors of the tracery. And an arrow, pointing to the tunnels beyond.

"They may be migrating," said Fet. "Pointing the way . . ."

Eph nodded, and followed Fet's gaze. The direction it indicated was southeast.

"My father used to tell me about these markings," said Fet. "Hobo speak—from when he first came to this country after the war. Chalk drawings indicating friendly and unfriendly houses—where you might get fed, find a bed, or even to warn others about a hostile homeowner. Throughout the years, I've seen similar signs in warehouses, in tunnels, cellars . . ."

"What does it mean?"

"I don't know the language." He looked around. "But it seems to be pointing that way. See if one of those phones has any battery left. One with a camera."

Eph rooted through the top of the pile, trying phones and discarding the dark ones. A pink Nokia with a glow-in-the-dark Hello Kitty charm winked to life in his hand. He tossed it to Fet.

Fet looked it over. "I never understood this fucking cat. The head is too big. How is it even a cat? Look at it. Is it sick with . . . with water inside it?"

"Hydrocephalic, you mean?" said Eph, wondering where this was coming from.

Fet ripped off the charm and tossed it away. "It's a jinx. Fucking cat. I hate that fucking cat."

He snapped a picture of the crescent glyph illuminated by indigo light, then videoed the entirety of the manic fresco, overwhelmed by the sight of it inside this gloomy chamber, haunted by the nature of its trespass—and mystified as to its meaning.

* * *

It was daylight when they emerged. Eph carried his sword and other equipment inside a baseball bag over his shoulder; Fet ported his weapons in a small rolling case that used to contain his exterminating tools and poisons. They were dressed for labor, and dirty from the tunnels beneath Ground Zero.

Wall Street was eerily quiet, the sidewalks nearly empty. Distant sirens wailed, begging a response that would not come. Black smoke was becoming a permanent fixture in the city sky.

The few pedestrians who did pass scurried by them quickly, with barely a nod. Some wore face masks, others shielded their noses and mouths with scarves—operating on misinformation about this mysterious "virus." Most shops and stores were closed—looted and empty or without power. They passed a market that was lit but unstaffed. People inside were taking what was left of the spoiled fruit in the stalls in front, or canned goods from the emptying shelves in back. Anything consumable. The drink cooler had already been raided, as had the refrigerated foods section. The cash register was cleaned out as well, because old habits die hard. But currency was hardly as valuable as water and food would be soon.

"Crazy," muttered Eph.

"At least some people still have power," said Fet. "Wait until their phones and laptops run dry, and they find they can't recharge. That's when the screaming starts."

Crosswalk signs changed symbols, going from the red hand to the white figure walking, but without crowds to cross. Manhattan without pedestrians was not Manhattan. Eph heard automobile horns out on the main avenues, but only an occasional taxi traversed the side streets—drivers hunched over steering wheels, fares sitting anxiously in the back.

They both paused at the next curb, out of habit, the crossing sign turning red. "Why now, do you think?" said Eph. "If they have been here so long, for centuries—what provoked this?"

Fet said, "His time horizon and ours, they are not the same. We measure our lives in days and years, by a calendar. He is a night creature. He has only the sky to concern him."

"The eclipse," said Eph suddenly. "He was waiting for that."

"Maybe it means something," said Fet. "Signifies something to him . . ."

Coming out of a station, a Transit Authority cop glanced at them, eyeing Eph.

"Shit." Eph looked away, but neither quickly nor casually enough. Even with the police forces breaking down, his face was on television a lot, and everybody was still watching, waiting to be told what to do.

As they moved on, the cop turned away. *It's just my paranoia,* Eph thought.

Around the corner, following precise instructions, the cop made a phone call.

Fet's Blog

HELLO THERE, WORLD.

Or what's left of it.

I used to think that there was nothing more useless than writing a blog.

I was unable to imagine any greater waste of time.

I mean, who cares what you have to say?

So I don't really know what this is.

But I need to do it.

I guess I have two reasons.

One is to set down my thoughts. To get them out onto this computer screen where I can see them and maybe make some sense out of all that is happening. Because what I have experienced in the past few days has changed me—literally—and I need to try and figure out who I am now.

The second reason?

Simple. Get out the truth. The truth of what is happening.

Who am I? I'm an exterminator by trade. So if you happen to live in one of the five boroughs of NYC, and you see a rat in your bathtub and you call pest control . . .

Yep. I'm the guy who shows up two weeks later.

You used to be able to leave that dirty job to me. Ridding pests. Eradicating vermin.

But not anymore.

A new infestation is spreading throughout the city, and into the world. A new breed of intruder. A pox upon the human race.

These creatures are nesting in your basement.

In your attic.

Your walls.

Now, here's the kicker.

With rats, mice, roaches—the best way to eliminate an infestation is to remove the food source.

Okay.

Only problem with that is that this new breed's food source?

That's right.

It's us.

You and me.

See, in case you haven't figured it out yet—we're in a shitload of trouble here.

Fairfield County, Connecticut

THE LOW-SLUNG BUILDING was one of a dozen at the end of the crumbling road, an office park that had been foundering even before the recession hit. It retained the sign of the previous tenant, R. L. Industries, a former armored car dispatcher and garage, and accordingly remained surrounded by a sturdy twelve-foot chain-link fence. Access was by key card through an electronic gate.

The garage half of the interior held the doctor's cream-colored Jaguar and a fleet of black vehicles befitting a dignitary's motorcade. The office half had been refitted into a small, private surgery dedicated to servicing one patient.

Eldritch Palmer lay in the recovery room, waking to the usual postoperative discomfort. He roused himself slowly but surely, having made this dark passage to returning consciousness many times before. His surgical team knew well the appropriate mix of sedatives and anesthesia. They never put him under deeply anymore. At his advanced age, it was too risky. And for Palmer, the less anesthesia used the faster he recovered.

He remained connected to machines testing the efficiency of his new liver. The donor had been a teenage Salvadorian runaway, tested to be disease-, drug-, and alcohol-free. A healthy, young, pinkish-brown organ, roughly triangular in shape, similar to an American football in size. Fresh off a jet plane, fewer than fourteen hours since harvesting, this allograft was, by Palmer's own count, his seventh liver. His body went through them the way coffee machines go through filters.

The liver, both the largest internal organ and the largest single gland in the human body, has many vital functions, including metabolism, glycogen storage, plasma synthesis, hormone production, and detoxification. Currently, there was no medical way to compensate for its absence in the body—which was most unfortunate for the reluctant Salvadorian donor.

Mr. Fitzwilliam, Palmer's nurse, bodyguard, and constant companion, stood in the corner, ever-vigilant in the manner of most ex-Marines. The surgeon entered, still wearing his mask, pulling on a fresh pair of gloves. The doctor was fastidious, ambitious, and, even by most surgeons' standards, incredibly wealthy.

He drew back the sheet. The newly stitched incision was a reopening of an older transplantation scar. Outwardly, Palmer's chest was a lumpy tableau of disfiguring scars. His interior torso was a hardened basket of failing organs. That was what the surgeon told him: "I am afraid your body cannot sustain any more tissue or organ allografts, Mr. Palmer. This is the end."

Palmer smiled. His body was a hive of other people's organs, and in that way he was not dissimilar from the Master, who was the embodiment of a hive of undead souls.

"Thank you, doctor. I understand." Palmer's voice was still raw from the breathing tube. "In fact, I suggest that you strike this surgery altogether. I know you are concerned about the AMA finding out about our techniques of organ harvesting, and I hereby release you from obligation. The fee you collect for this procedure will be your last. I will require no further medical intervention—not ever."

The surgeon's eyes remained uncertain. Eldritch Palmer, a sick man for nearly all his life, possessed an uncanny will to live: a fierce and unnatural survival instinct the likes of which the surgeon had never before encountered. Was he finally succumbing to his ultimate fate?

No matter. The surgeon was relieved, and grateful. His retirement had been planned for some time now, and everything was arranged. It was a blessing to be free of all obligations at such a tumultuous time as this. He only hoped the flights to Honduras were still in operation. And burning down this building would draw no inquiries in the wake of so much civil unrest.

All this the doctor swallowed with a polite smile. He withdrew under Mr. Fitzwilliam's steely gaze.

Palmer rested his eyes. He let his mind go back to the Master's solar exposure, perpetrated by that old fool, Setrakian. Palmer assessed this development in the only terms he understood: What did it mean for him?

It only sped up the timeline, which, in turn, expedited his imminent deliverance.

At long last, his day was nearly at hand.

Setrakian. Did defeat indeed taste bitter? Or was it more akin to ashes on the tongue?

Palmer had never known defeat—*would* never know defeat. And how many can say that?

Like a stone in the middle of a swift river, stood Setrakian. Foolishly and proudly believing he was disrupting the flow—when, in fact, the river was predictably running full-speed right around him.

The futility of humans. It all starts out with such promise, doesn't it? And yet all ends so predictably.

His thoughts turned to the Palmer Foundation. It was indeed expected among the super-rich that each of the world's wealthiest endow a charitable organization in his own name. This, his one and only philanthropic foundation, had used its ample resources to transport and treat two full busloads of children afflicted by the recent occultation of the Earth. Children struck blind during that rare celestial event—either as a result of peeking at the eclipsed sun without proper optical protection, or else due to an unfortunate defect in the lenses of a batch of child-size safety glasses. The faulty glasses had been traced back to a plant in China, the trail running cold at an empty lot in Taipei . . .

No expense was to be spared in the rehabilitation and re-education of these poor souls, his foundation pledged. And indeed, Palmer meant it.

The Master had demanded it so.

Pearl Street

EPH FELT THAT they were being followed as they crossed the street. Fet, on the other hand, was focused on the rats. The displaced rodents scurried from door to door and along the sunny gutter, evidently in a state of panic and chaos.

"Look up there," said Fet.

What Eph thought were pigeons perched on the ledges were, in fact, rats. Looking down, watching Eph and Fet as though waiting to see what they would do. Their presence was instructive as a barometer of the vampire infestation spreading underground, driving rats from their nests. Something about the animal vibrations the *strigoi* gave off, or else their manifestly evil presence, repelled other forms of life.

"There must be a nest nearby," said Fet.

They neared a bar, and Eph felt a thirsty tug at

the back of his throat. He doubled back and tried the door, finding it unlocked. An ancient bar, established more than 150 years ago—the oldest continually operating ale house in New York City, bragged the sign—but no patrons, and no bartender. The only disruption to the silence was the low chatter of a television in a high corner, playing the news.

They walked to the back bar, which was darker, and just as empty. Half-consumed mugs of beer sat on the tables, and a few chairs still had coats hanging off them. When the party ended here, it had ended abruptly and all at once.

Eph checked the bathrooms—the men's room containing great and ancient urinals ending in a trough beneath the floor—and found them predictably empty.

He came back out, his boots scuffing the sawdust on the floor. Fet had set down his case and pulled out a chair, resting his legs.

Eph stepped behind the back bar. No liquor bottles or blenders or buckets of ice—just beer taps, with shelves of ten-ounce glass mugs waiting below. The place served only beer. No liquor, which was what Eph wanted. Only its own branded brew, available in either light or dark ale. The old taps were for show, but the newer ones flowed smoothly. Eph poured two dark draughts. "Here's to . . . ?"

Fet got to his feet and walked to the bar, taking up one of the mugs. "Killing bloodsuckers."

Eph drained half his mug. "Looks like people cleared out of here in a hurry."

"Last call," said Fet, swiping the foam off his thick upper lip. "Last call all over town."

A voice from the television got their attention, and they walked into the front room. A reporter was doing a live shot from a town near Bronxville, the hometown of one of the four survivors of Flight 753. Smoke darkened the sky behind him, the news crawl reading, BRONXVILLE RIOTS CONTINUE.

Fet reached up to change the channel. Wall Street was reeling from consumer fear, the threat of an outbreak greater than the H1N1 flu, and a rash of disappearances among their own brokers. Traders were shown sitting immobilized while the market averages plummeted.

On NY1, traffic was the focus, every exit out of Manhattan congested with people fleeing the island ahead of a rumored quarantine. Air and rail travel were overbooked, the airports and train station scenes of sheer chaos.

Eph heard a helicopter overhead. A chopper was probably the only easy way in or out of Manhattan now. If you had your own helipad. Like Eldritch Palmer.

Eph found an old-school, hard-wired telephone behind the bar. He got a scratchy dial tone and patiently used the rotary face to dial Setrakian's.

It rang through, and Nora answered. "How's Zack?" Eph asked, before she could speak.

"Better. He was really flipped out for a while."

"She never came back?"

"No. Setrakian ran her off the roof."

"Off the roof? Good Christ." Eph felt sick. He

grabbed a clean mug and couldn't pour another beer fast enough. "Where's Z now?"

"Upstairs. You want me to get him?"

"No. Better if I talk to him face-to-face when I get back."

"I think you're right. Did you destroy the coffin?"

"No," said Eph. "It was gone."

"Gone?" she said.

"Apparently he's not badly injured. Not slowed down much at all. And—this is weird, but there were some strange drawings on the wall down there, spray paint—"

"What do you mean, someone putting up graffiti?"

Eph patted the phone in his pocket, reassuring himself that the pink phone was still there. "I got some video. I really don't know what to make of it." He pulled the phone away for a moment to swallow more beer. "I'll tell you, though. The city—it's eerie. Quiet."

"Not here," said Nora. "There's a little bit of a lull now that it's dawn—but it won't last. The sun doesn't seem to scare them as much now. Like they're becoming bolder."

"That's exactly what it is," said Eph. "They're learning, becoming smarter. We have to get out of there. Today."

"Setrakian was just saying that. Because of Kelly."

"Because she knows where we are now?"

"Because she knows—that means the Master knows."

Eph pressed his hand against his closed eyes, pushing back on his headache. "Okay."

"Where are you now?"

"Financial District, near the Ferry Loop station." He didn't mention that he was in a bar. "Fet has a line on a bigger car. We're going to get that and head back soon."

"Just—please get back here in one human piece."

"That's our plan."

He hung up, and went rooting underneath the bar. He was looking for a container to hold more beer, which he needed for the descent back underground. Something other than a glass mug. He found an old, leather-jacketed flask, and, in brushing the dust off the brass cap, discovered a bottle of good vintage brandy behind it. No dust on the brandy: probably there for a quick nip for the barkeep to break the monotony of the ale. He rinsed out the flask and was filling it carefully over a small sink when he heard a knock at the door.

He came around the bar fast, heading for his weapon bag before realizing: vampires don't knock. He continued past Fet to the door, cautiously, looking through the window and seeing Dr. Everett Barnes, the director of the Centers for Disease Control and Prevention. The old country doctor was not wearing his admiral's uniform—the CDC was originally born of the U.S. Navy—but rather an ivory-on-white suit, the jacket unbuttoned. He looked as though he had rushed away from a late breakfast.

Eph could view the immediate street area behind him, and Barnes was apparently alone, at least for the moment. Eph unlocked the door and pulled it open.

"Ephraim," said Barnes.

Eph grabbed him by his lapel and hauled him inside fast, locking up again. "You," he said, checking the street again. "Where are the rest?"

Director Barnes pulled away from Eph, readjusting his jacket. "They are on orders to keep well back. But they will be here soon, make no mistake about that. I insisted that I needed a few minutes alone with you."

"Jesus," said Eph, checking the rooftops across the street before backing away from the front windows. "How did they get you here so fast?"

"It is a priority that I speak to you. No one wants to harm you, Ephraim. This was all done at my behest."

Eph turned away from him, heading back to the bar. "Maybe you only think so."

"We need you to come in," said Barnes, following him. "I need you, Ephraim. I know this now."

"Look," said Eph, reaching the bar and turning. "Maybe you understand what's going on, and maybe you don't. Maybe you're part of it, I don't know. You might not even know. But there is someone behind this, someone very powerful, and if I go anywhere with you now, it will certainly result in my incapacitation or death. Or worse."

"I am eager to listen to you, Ephraim. Whatever you have to say. I stand before you as a man admitting his mistake. I know now that we are in the grip of something altogether devastating and otherworldly."

"Not otherworldly. This-worldly." Eph capped his brandy flask.

Fet was behind Barnes. "How long until they come in?" he asked.

"Not long," said Barnes, unsure of the big exterminator in the dirty jumpsuit. Barnes returned his attention to Eph, and the flask. "Should you be drinking now?"

"Now more than ever," said Eph. "Help yourself if you want. I recommend the dark ale."

"Look, I know you've been put through a lot—"

"What happens to *me* doesn't really matter, Everett. This isn't about me, so any appeals to my ego won't get you anywhere. What I *am* concerned about are these half-truths—or, should I say, outright lies—being issued under the auspices of the CDC. Are you no longer serving the public now, Everett? Just your government?"

Director Barnes winced. "Necessarily both."

"Weak," said Eph. "Inept. Even criminal."

"This is why I need you to come in, Ephraim. I need your eyewitness experience, your expertise—"

"It's too late! Can't you at least see that?"

Barnes backed off a bit, keeping an eye on Fet because Fet made him nervous. "You were right about Bronxville. We've closed it off."

"Closed it off?" said Fet. "How?"

"A wire fence."

Eph laughed bitterly. "A wire fence? Jesus,

Everett. This is exactly what I mean. You're reacting to the *public perception* of the virus, rather than the threat itself. Reassuring them with fences? With a *symbol*? They will tear those fences apart—"

"Then tell me. Tell me what I need. What *you* need."

"Start with destroying the corpses. That is step number one."

"Destroy the . . . ? You know I can't do that."

"Then nothing else you do matters. You have to send in a military team and sweep through that place and eliminate every single carrier. Then expand that operation south, into the city here, and all across Brooklyn and the Bronx . . ."

"You're talking mass killing. Think about the visuals—"

"Think about the *reality*, Everett. I am a doctor, same as you. But this is a new world now."

Fet drifted away, back toward the front, keeping an eye on the street. Eph said, "They don't want you to bring me in to help. They want you to bring me in so they can neutralize me and the people I know. This"—he crossed to his weapons bag, drawing a silver sword—"is my scalpel now. The only way to heal these creatures is to release them—and yes, that means wholesale slaughter. Not doctoring. You want to help—to really help? Then get on TV and tell them that. Tell them the truth."

Barnes looked at Fet in the front. "And who is this one with you now? I expected to see you with Dr. Martinez."

Something about the way Barnes said Nora's

name struck Eph as odd. But he could not pursue it. Fet came back quickly from the front windows.

"Here they come," said Fet.

Eph ventured near enough to see vans pulling up, closing off the street in either direction. Fet passed him, grabbing Barnes by the shoulder and walking him to a table in back, sitting him in the corner. Eph slung his baseball bag over his shoulder and ported Fet's case to him.

"Please," said Barnes. "I implore you. Both of you. I can protect you."

"Listen," said Fet. "You just officially became a hostage, so shut the fuck up." To Eph, he said: "Now what? How do we hold them off? UVC light doesn't work on the FBI."

Eph looked around the old ale house for answers. The pictures and ephemera of a century and a half, hanging on the walls and cluttering the shelves behind the bar. Portraits of Lincoln, Garfield, McKinley, and a bust of JFK—all assassinated presidents. Nearby, among such curios as a musket, a shaving-cream mug, and framed obituaries, hung a small silver dagger.

Near it, a sign: WE WERE HERE BEFORE YOU WERE BORN.

Eph rushed behind the bar. He kicked aside the sawdust over the bull-nose ring latch embedded in the worn wooden floor.

Fet, appearing at his side, helped him raise the trapdoor.

The odor told them everything they needed to know. Ammonia. Pungent and recent.

Director Barnes, still in his seat in the corner, said, "They'll only come in after you."

"Judging by the smell—I wouldn't recommend it," said Fet, starting down first.

"Everett," said Eph, switching on his Luma lamp before going down. "In case there is any lingering ambiguity, let me be perfectly clear now. I quit."

Eph followed Fet to the bottom, his lamp illuminating the supply area beneath the bar in ethereal indigo. Fet reached up to close the door overhead.

"Leave it," muttered Eph. "If he's as dirty as I think he is, he's running for the door already."

Fet did, the hatch remaining open.

The ceiling was low, and the detritus of many decades—old kegs and barrels, a few broken chairs, stacks of empty glass racks, and an old industrial dishwasher—narrowed the passageway. Fet adjusted thick rubber bands around his ankles and jacket cuffs—a trick from his days baiting roach-infested apartments, learned the hard way. He handed some to Eph. "For worms," he said, zipping his jacket tight.

Eph crossed the stone floor, pushing open a side door leading to an old, warm ice room. It was empty.

Next came a wooden door with an old, oval knob. The floor dust before it was disturbed in the shape of a fan. Fet nodded to him, and Eph yanked it open.

You don't hesitate. You don't think. Eph had learned that. You never give them time to group up and anticipate, because it is in their makeup that one of them will sacrifice itself in order that the others might have a chance at you. Facing stingers that can reach five or six feet, and their extraordinary night vision, you never, ever stop moving until every last monster is destroyed.

The neck was their vulnerable point—same as their prey's throat was to them. Sever the spinal column and you destroy the body and the being that inhabits it. A significant amount of white-blood loss achieves the same end, though blood-letting is much more dangerous, as the capillary worms that escape live on outside the body, seeking new human bodies to invade. Why Fet liked to band up his cuffs.

Eph destroyed the first two in the manner that had proved most effective: using the UVC lamp like a torch to repel the beast, isolating and trapping them against a wall, then closing in with the sword for the coup de grâce. Weapons made of silver do wound them, and cause whatever constitutes the vampire equivalent of human pain—and ultraviolet light burns through their DNA like flame.

Fet used the nail gun, pumping silver brads into their faces to blind or otherwise disorient them, then running through their distended throats. Loosened worms slithered across the wet floor. Eph killed some of the worms with his UVC light, while others met their fate beneath the hard treads of Fet's boots. Fet, after stomping a few of them, scooped them into a small jar from his case. "For the old man," he said, before continuing on with his slaying.

They heard a multitude of footsteps and voices in the bar above them as they pressed on into the next room.

One came at Eph from the side—still wearing a bartending apron—its eyes wide and hungry. Eph slashed at it backhandedly, driving the creature back with the lamp light. Eph was learning to ignore his physician's inclination toward mercy. The vampire gnashed pitifully in a corner as Eph closed in, finishing it off.

Two others, maybe three, had taken off through the next door as soon as they saw the indigo light coming. A handful remained, crouched beneath broken shelves, ready to attack.

Fet came alongside Eph, lamp in hand. Eph started toward the vampires, but Fet caught his arm. Whereas Eph was breathing hard, the exterminator proceeded in a businesslike manner, focused without distress.

"Wait," said Fet. "Leave them for Barnes's FBI buddies."

Eph, seeing the advantage of Fet's idea, backed off, still with his lamp trained on them. "Now what?"

"Those others ran. There's a way out."

Eph looked at the next door. "You better be right," he said.

Fet took the lead belowground, following the trail of dried urine fluorescing underneath the

Luma lamps. The rooms gave way to a series of cellars, connected by old, hand-dug tunnels. The ammonia markings went in many different directions, Fet selecting one, turning off at a junction.

"I like this," he said, stamping muck off his boots. "Just like rat hunting, following the trail. The UV light makes it easy."

"But how do they know these routes?"

"They've been busy. Exploring, foraging. You never heard of the Volstead Grid?"

"Volstead? Like the Volstead Act? Prohibition?"

"Restaurants, bars, speakeasies, they had to open up their cellars, go underground. This is a city that just keeps building over itself. Combine the old cellars and houses under there with the tunnels, aqueducts, and old utility pipes—and some say you can move block to block, neighborhood to neighborhood, solely underground, between any two points in the city."

"Bolivar's place," said Eph, remembering the rock star who had been one of the four survivors of Flight 753. His building was an old bootlegger's house, with a secret gin cellar that linked to the subway tunnels below. Eph checked behind them as they passed a side tunnel. "How do you know where you're going?"

Fet pointed to another hobo signal scratched into the stone, probably with one of the creature's hardened talon nails. "We're on to something here," he said. "That's all I know for sure. But I bet the Ferry Loop Station isn't more than a block or two away."

Nazareth, Pennsylvania

AUGUSTIN . . .

Augustin Elizalde got to his feet. He stood in a stew of absolute darkness. A palpable inky blackness without a hint of light. Like space with no stars. He blinked his eyes to make certain that they were open—and they were. No change.

Was this death? No place could be darker.

Must be. He was fucking dead.

Or—maybe they had turned him. Was he a vampire now, his body taken over, but this old part of him shut away in the darkness of his mind, like a prisoner in an attic? Maybe the coolness he felt and the hardness of the floor beneath his feet were just compensatory tricks of his brain. He was walled up forever inside his own head.

He crouched a bit, trying to establish his existence through movement and sensory impression. He grew dizzy due to the lack of a visual focal point, and set his feet wider apart. He reached up, jumping, but could feel no ceiling above him.

An occasional faint breeze rippled his shirt. It smelled like soil. Like earth.

He was underground. Buried alive.

Augustin . . .

Again. His mother's voice calling to him as in a dream.

"Mama?"

His voice doubled back on him in a startling echo. He remembered her as he had left her: sitting in the bottom of her bedroom closet, under a great pile of clothes. Staring up at him with the leering hunger of a newly turned *them*.

Vampires, the old man said.

Gus turned, trying to guess in which direction the voice might have originated. He had nothing else to do but follow this voice.

He walked to a stone wall, feeling his way along its smooth and slowly curving face. His palms remained sore where the glass had cut him—the shard he had wielded in the murder (no—the *destruction*) of his brother-turned-vampire. He stopped to feel his wrists, and realized the handcuffs he had been wearing at the time of his escape from police custody—the ones whose chain the hunters had split—were now gone.

Those hunters. They had turned out to be vampires themselves, appearing on that street in Morningside Heights and battling the other vampires like two sides in a gang war. But the hunters were well equipped. They had weapons, and they were coordinated. They drove cars. They weren't just the bloodthirsty attack drones like the ones Gus had faced and destroyed.

The last thing he remembered was them throwing Gus into the back of an SUV. But—why him?

Another puff of wind, like Mother Nature's last breath, brushed against his face, and he followed it—hoping he was moving in the right direction. The wall ended at a sharp corner. He felt for the opposite side, his left, and found it the same: ending at a corner, with a gap in between. Just like a doorway.

Gus stepped through, and the new echo of his footsteps told him that this room was wider and higher-ceilinged than the rest. A faint smell here, familiar to him somehow. Trying to place it.

He got it. The cleaning solution he'd had to use in lockup, on maintenance detail. It was ammonia. Not enough to singe the inside of his nose.

Then something started to happen. He thought his mind was playing tricks, but then realized that, yes, light was coming to the room. The slowness of the illumination, and the general uncertainty of the situation, terrified him. Two tripod lamps set wide apart, near the far walls, were coming up gradually, diluting the thick blackness.

Gus drew his arms in tight, in the manner of the mixed-martial-arts fighters he watched on the Internet. The lights kept brightening, though so gradually that the wattage barely registered. But his pupils were so widely dilated by the darkness, his retina so exposed, that any light source would have caused a reaction.

He didn't see it at first. The being was right in front of him, no more than ten or fifteen feet away, but its head and limbs were so pale and still and smooth that his eyes read them as part of the walls of rock.

The only thing that stood out was a pair of symmetrical dark holes. Not black holes, but almost black.

The deepest red. Blood red.

If they were eyes, they did not blink. Nor did they stare. They looked upon Gus with a remarkable lack of passion. These were eyes as indifferent as red stones. Blood-sodden eyes that had seen it all.

Gus glimpsed the outline of a robe on the being's body, blending into the darkness like a cavity within the cavity. The being stood tall, if he was making it out correctly. But the stillness of this thing was deathlike. Gus did not move.

"What is this?" he said, his voice coming out a little funny, betraying his fear. "You think you're eating Mexican tonight? You wanna think twice about that. How 'bout you come and choke on it, bitch."

It radiated such silence and stillness that Gus might have been looking at some clothed statue. Its skull was hairless and smooth all over, lacking the cartilage of ears. Now Gus was aware of something, hearing—or, rather, feeling—a vibration like humming.

"Well?" he said, addressing the expressionless eyes. "What you waiting for? You like to play with your food before you eat it?" He pulled his fists in closer to his face. "Not this fucking *chalupa*, you undead piece of shit."

Something other than movement drew his attention to the right—and he saw that there was another one. Standing there like part of the stone wall, a shade shorter than the first one, eyes shaped differently but similarly emotionless.

And then, to the left—gradually, to Gus's eyes—a third.

Gus, who was not unfamiliar with court-rooms, felt like he was appearing before three alien judges inside a stone chamber. He was going out of his mind, but his reaction was to keep shooting off his mouth. To keep putting up the gangbanger front. The judges he had faced called it "contempt." Gus called it "coping." What he did when he felt looked down upon. When he felt he was being treated not as a unique human being but as an inconvenience, an obstacle dropped in someone's way.

We will be brief.

Gus's hands shot up to his temples. Not his ears: the voice was somehow *inside* his head. Coming from that same part of his brain where his own interior monologue originated—as though some pirate radio station had started broadcasting on his signal.

You are Augustin Elizalde.

He gripped his head but the voice was tight in there. No off switch.

"Yeah, I know who the fuck I am. Who the fuck are you? *What* the fuck are you? And how did you get inside my—"

You are not here as sustenance. We have plenty of livestock on hand for the snow season.

Livestock? "Oh, you mean people?" Gus had heard occasional yells, anguished voices echoing through the caves, but imagined they were cries in his dreams.

Free-range husbandry has suited our needs for thou-sands of years. Dumb animals make for plentiful food. On occasion, one shows unusual resourcefulness.

Gus barely followed that, wanting them to get to the point. "So—what, you're saying you're not going to try to turn me into . . . one of you?"

Our bloodline is pristine and privileged. To enter into our heritage is a gift. Entirely unique and very, very expensive.

They weren't making any sense to Gus. "If you're not going to drink my blood—then what the hell do you want?"

We have a proposal.

"A proposal?" Gus banged on the side of his head as though it were a malfunctioning appliance. "I guess I'm fucking listening—unless I have a choice."

We need a daylight serf. A hunter. We are a nocturnal race of beings, you are diurnal.

"Diurnal?"

Your endogenous circadian rhythm corresponds directly to the light-dark cycle of what you call a twenty-four-hour day. Your kind's inbred chronobiology is acclimated to this planet's celestial timetable, in reverse of ours. You are a sun creature.

"Fucking what?"

We need someone who can move about freely during daylight hours. One who can withstand sun exposure, and, in fact, use its power, as well as any other weapons at his disposal, to massacre the unclean.

"Massacre the unclean? You are vampires, right? Are you saying you want me killing your own kind?"

Not our kind. This unclean strain spreading so promiscuously through your people—it is a scourge. It is out of control.

"What did you expect?"

We had no part in this. Before you, stand beings of great honor and discretion. This contagion represents the violation of a truce—an equilibrium—that has lasted for centuries. This is a direct affront.

Gus stepped back a few inches. He actually thought he was starting to understand now. "Somebody's trying to move in on your block."

We do not breed in the same random, chaotic manner as your kind. Ours is a process of careful consideration.

"You're picky eaters."

We eat what we want. Food is food. We dispose of it when we are satiated.

A laugh rose inside Gus's chest, nearly choking him. Talking about people like they were three for a dollar at the corner market.

You find that humorous?

"No. The opposite. That's why I'm laughing."

When you consume an apple, do you throw away the core? Or do you conserve the seeds for planting more trees?

"I guess I throw it away."

And a plastic receptacle? When you've emptied its contents?

"Fine, I get it. You throw back your pints of blood and then toss away the human bottle. Here's what I want to know. Why me?"

Because you appear capable.

"How you figure that?"

Your criminal record, for one. You came to our attention through your arrest for murder in Manhattan.

The fat, naked guy rampaging through Times Square. The guy had attacked a family there, and

at the time Gus was like, "Not in my city, freak."
Now, of course, he wished he had stayed back
like all the rest.

*Then you escaped police custody, slaying more un-
cleans in the process.*

Gus frowned. "That 'unclean' was my compa-
dre. How you know all this, living down here in
this shithole?"

*Be assured that we are connected with the human
world at its uppermost levels. But, if balance is to be
maintained, we cannot afford exposure—precisely
what this unclean strain threatens us with now. That is
where you come in.*

"A gang war. That, I understand. But you left
out something super-fucking important. Like—
why the fuck should I help you?"

Three reasons.

"I'm counting. They better be good ones."

The first is, you will leave this room alive.

"I'll give you that one."

*The second is, your success in this endeavor will
enrich you beyond that which you ever thought possible.*

"Hmm. I don't know. I can count pretty high."

The third . . . is right behind you.

Gus turned. He saw a hunter first, one of the
badass vamps who had grabbed him off the street.
Its head was cowled inside a black hoodie, its red
eyes glowing.

Next to the hunter was a vampire with that
look of distant hunger now familiar to Gus. She
was short and heavy, with tangled black hair,
wearing a torn housedress, the upper front of her

throat bulging with the interior architecture of the vampire stinger.

At the base of the stitched V of her dress collar was a highly stylized, black-and-red crucifix, a tattoo she said she regretted getting in her youth but which must have looked pretty fucking boss at the time, and which, since his youngest days, had always impressed Gusto, no matter what she said.

The vampire was his mother. Her eyes were blindfolded with a dark rag. Gus could see the throbbing of her throat, the want of her stinger.

She senses you. But her eyes must remain covered. Within her resides the will of our enemy. He sees through her. Hears through her. We cannot keep her in this chamber for long.

Gus's eyes filled with angry tears. The sorrow ached in him, manifested in rage. Since about age eleven, he had done nothing but dishonor her. And now here she was before him: a beast, an undead monster.

Gus turned back to face the others. This fury surged within him, but here he was powerless, and he knew it.

The third is, you get to release her.

Dry sobs came up like sorrowful belches. He was sickened by this situation, appalled by it, and yet . . .

He turned back around. She was as good as kidnapped. Taken hostage by this "unclean" strain of vampire they kept talking about.

"Mama," he said. Although she listened, she showed no change of expression.

Slaying his brother, Crispin, had been easy, because of the longstanding bad feelings between them. Because Crispin was an addict and even more of a failure than Gus. Doing Crispin through the neck with that shard of broken glass had been efficiency in action: family therapy and garbage disposal rolled into one. The rage he accumulated through decades had evaporated with every slash.

But delivering his *madre* from this curse, that would be an act of love.

Gus's mother was removed from the chamber, but the hunter stayed behind. Gus looked back at the three, seeing them better now. Awful in their stillness. They never moved.

We will provide you with anything you need to achieve this task. Capital support is not an issue, as we have amassed vast fortunes of human treasure through time.

Those who received the gift of eternity had paid fortunes over the centuries. Within their vaults, the Ancient Ones held Mesopotamian coils of silver, Byzantine coins, sovereigns, Deutsche marks. The currency mattered nothing to them. Shells to trade with the natives. "So—you want me to fetch for you—is that it?"

Mr. Quinlan will provide you with anything you need. Anything. He is our best hunter. Efficient and loyal. In many respects, unique. Your only restriction is secrecy. Concealment of our existence is paramount. We leave it to you to recruit other hunters such as yourself. Invisible and unknown, yet skilled at killing.

Gus bridled, feeling the pull of his mother behind him. An outlet for his wrath: maybe this was just what he needed.

His lips pursed into an angry smile. He needed manpower. He needed killers.

He knew exactly where to go next.

IRT South Ferry Inner Loop Station

FET, WITH ONLY one false turn, led them to a tunnel that connected to the abandoned South Ferry Loop Station. Dozens of phantom subway stations dot the IRT, the IND, and the BMT systems. You don't see them on the maps anymore, though they can be glimpsed through in-service subway car windows on active rails—if you know when and where to look.

The underground climate was more humid here, a dampness in the ground soil, the walls slick and weeping.

The glowing trail of *strigoi* waste became more scarce here. Fet looked around, puzzled. He knew that the route down Broadway was part of the city's original subway project, South Ferry having opened for commuters in 1905. The underwater tunnel to Brooklyn opened three years later.

The original mosaic tiling featuring the station initials, SF, still stood, high on the wall, near an incongruously modern sign—

NO TRAINS STOP HERE

—as if anyone would make that mistake. Eph moved into a small maintenance bay, scanning with his Luma.

Out of the darkness, a voice cackled, "Are you IRT?"

Eph smelled the man before he saw him. The figure emerged from a nearby alcove stuffed with ripped and soiled mattresses—a toothless scarecrow of a man dressed in multiple layers of shirts, coats, and pants. His body scent patiently distilled and aged through all of them.

"No," said Fet, taking over. "We're not here rousting anybody."

The man looked them over, rendering a snap judgment as to their trustworthiness. "Name's Cray-Z," he said. "You from up top?"

"Sure," said Eph.

"What's it like? I'm one of the last ones here."

"Last ones?" said Eph. He noticed, for the first time, the shabby outline of a few tents and cardboard housings. After a moment, a few more spectral figures emerged. The "Mole People," denizens of the urban abyss, the fallen, the disgraced, the disenfranchised, the "broken windows" of the Giuliani era. This was where they eventually found their way to, the city below, where it remained warm 24/7, even in the dead of winter. With luck and experience, one could camp at a site for as many as six months at a time, even more. Away from the busier stations, some resided for years without ever seeing a maintenance crew.

Cray-Z looked at Eph with his head turned to favor his one good eye. The other one was covered in granulated cataracts. "That's right. Most all the colony is gone—just like the rats. Yeah, man. Vanished, leaving them fine valuables behind."

He gestured at discarded piles of junk: ragged sleeping bags, muddy shoes, some coats. Fet felt a pang, knowing that these articles represented the sum total of the worldly possessions of the recently departed.

Cray-Z smiled a vacant smile. "Unusual, man. Downright spooky."

Fet remembered something he had read in *National Geographic,* or maybe watched one night on the History channel: the story of a colony of settlers in the pre-America era—in Roanoke, maybe—who vanished one day. Over a hundred people, gone, leaving behind all of their belongings but no clues to their sudden and mysterious departure, nothing except two cryptic carvings: the word CROATOAN written into a post on their fort, and the letters CRO whittled into the bark of a nearby tree.

Fet looked again at the mosaic SF tiled onto the high wall.

"I know you," said Eph, keeping a polite distance from the reeking Cray-Z. "I've seen you around—I mean, up there." He pointed toward the surface. "You carry one of those signs. GOD IS WATCHING YOU, or something like that."

Cray-Z smiled a mostly toothless smile and went and pulled out his hand-drawn placard, proud of his celebrity status. GOD IS WATCHING YOU!!! in bright red, with three exclamation points for emphasis.

Cray-Z was indeed a semi-delusional zealot. Down here, he was an outcast among outcasts. He had lived underground as long as anyone—maybe longer. He claimed that he could get anywhere in the city without surfacing—and yet he apparently lacked the ability to urinate without splashing the toes of his shoes.

Cray-Z moved alongside the tracks, motioning for Eph and Fet to follow. He ducked inside a tarp-and-pallet shack, where old, nibbled extension cords wound away up into the roof, wired into some hidden source of electricity on the great city grid.

It had begun to drizzle lightly within the tunnel, weeping ceiling pipes wetting the dirt, their water splattering onto Cray-Z's tarp and running down into a waiting Gatorade bottle.

Cray-Z emerged carrying an old promotional cutout of former New York City Mayor Ed Koch, flashing his trademark "How'm I Doing?" smile. "Here," he said, handing the life-sized photo to Eph. "Hold this."

Cray-Z then walked them to the far tunnel, pointing down its tracks.

"Right into there," he said. "That's where they all went."

"Who? The people?" said Eph, setting Mayor Koch down next to him. "They went into the tunnel?"

Cray-Z laughed. "No. Not just the tunnel, shithead. Down *there*. Where the pipes at the curve go under the East River, across to Governor's

Island, then over to mainland Brooklyn at Red Hook. That's where they *took* them."

"Took them?" said Eph, a chill trickling down his spine. "Who—who took them?"

Just then, a track signal lit up nearby. Eph jumped back. "This track still active?"

Fet said, "The 5 train still turns around on the inner loop."

Cray-Z spat onto the tracks. "Man knows his trains."

Light grew inside the space as the train approached, brightening the old station, bringing it briefly to life. Mayor Koch shook under Eph's hand.

"You watch real close, now," said Cray-Z. "No blinking!" He covered his blind eye and smiled his mostly toothless smile.

The train thundered past them, taking the turn a little faster than usual. The cars were nearly vacant inside, maybe one or two people visible through the windows, here and there a solitary straphanger. Abovegrounders just passing through.

Cray-Z gripped Eph's forearm as the end of the train approached. "There—*right there*—"

In the flickering light of the passing train, Fet and Eph saw something on the rear exterior of the final car. A cluster of figures—of bodies, people—flat against the outside of the train. Clinging to it like remoras riding a steel shark.

"You see that?" exulted Cray-Z. "You see 'em all? The Other People."

Eph shook loose of Cray-Z's grip, taking a few steps forward away from him and Mayor Koch, the train finishing its loop and dwindling into darkness, the light leaving the tunnel like water down a drain.

Cray-Z started hustling back to his shack. "Somebody has to do something, right? You guys just decided it for me. These are the dark angels at the end of time. They'll snatch us all if we let 'em."

Fet took a few lumbering steps after the receding train, before stopping and looking back at Eph. "The tunnels. It's how they get across. They can't go over moving water, right? Not unassisted."

Eph was right there with him. "But *under* the water. Nothing stops them from that."

"Progress," said Fet. "This is the trouble progress gets us in. What do you call it—when you figure out you can get away with shit that nobody made up a specific rule for?"

"A loophole," said Eph.

"Exactly. This, right here?" Fet opened his arms, gesturing at their surroundings. "We just discovered one giant gaping loophole."

The Coach

THE LUXURY COACH bus departed New Jersey's St. Lucia's Home for the Blind in the early afternoon, headed for an exclusive academy in Upstate New York.

The driver, with his corny stories and an entire catalog of knock-knock jokes, made the journey fun for his passengers, some sixty nervous children between the ages of seven and twelve. Their cases had been culled from emergency-room reports throughout the tristate area. These children were recently visually impaired—all had been accidentally blinded by the recent lunar occultation—and, for many, this was their first trip without a parent present.

Their scholarships, all offered and provided by the Palmer Foundation, included this orientation-like camp outing, an immersive retreat in adaptive techniques for the newly blind. Their chaperones—nine young adult graduates of St. Lucia's—were each legally blind, meaning their central visual acuity rated 20/200 or less, though they had some residual light perception. The children in their care were all clinically NLP, or "no light perception," meaning totally blind. The driver was the only sighted person on board.

The traffic was slow in many spots, due to the jam-ups surrounding Greater New York, but the driver kept the children entertained with riddles and banter. At other times, he narrated the ride, or described the interesting things he could see out the window, or invented details in order to make the mundane interesting. He was a longtime employee of St. Lucia's, who didn't mind playing the clown. He knew that one secret to unlocking the potential of these traumatized children, and opening their hearts to the challenges ahead, was to feed their imagination and involve and engage them.

"Knock-knock."

Who's there?

"Disguise."

Disguise who?

"Disguise jokes are killing me."

The stop at McDonald's went well, all things considered, except that the Happy Meal toy was a hologram card. The driver sat apart from the group, watching the youngsters finding their French fries with tentative hands, having not yet learned to "clock" their meal for ease of consumption. At the same time, unlike the majority of blind children who were born sight-impaired, McDonald's had visual meaning for them, and they seemed to find comfort in the smooth plastic swivel chairs and oversize drinking straws.

Back on the road, the three-hour ride stretched into double that amount of time. The chaperones led the children singing in rounds, then broadcast some audiobooks on the overhead video screens. A number of the younger children, their biological clocks thrown off by blindness, dozed on and off.

The chaperones perceived the change in light quality through the coach windows, aware of darkness falling outside. The coach moved more swiftly as they got into New York State—until all at once they felt it decelerate suddenly, enough so that stuffed animals and drink cups fell to the floor.

The coach pulled to the side and stopped.

"What is it?" asked the lead chaperone, a twenty-four-year-old assistant teacher named Joni, sitting closest to the front of the bus.

"Don't know . . . something strange. Just sit tight. I'll be right back."

Then the driver was gone, but the chaperones were too busy to worry—anytime the coach stopped, hands went up for assistance to the restroom in back.

Some ten minutes later, the driver returned. He started up the bus without a word, despite the fact that the chaperones were still supervising bathroom trips. Joni's request to him to wait was ignored, but the kids were eventually helped back to their seats, and everyone was okay.

The coach rolled on quietly from there. The audio program was not continued. The driver's banter ceased, and, in fact, he refused to respond to any questions Joni asked, seated right behind him in the first row. She grew alarmed, but decided she must not let the others sense her concern. She told herself that the coach was still moving properly, they were traveling at an appropriate rate of speed, and anyway they had to be close to their destination by now.

Some time later, the coach turned onto a dirt road, waking everyone up. Then it rolled onto even rougher ground, everyone holding on, drinks spilling into laps as the bus bumped along. They endured this shaking for one full minute—until the bus abruptly stopped.

The driver turned off the engine and they heard the door fold open with a pneumatic hiss.

He departed without a word, his keys jingling faintly into the distance.

Joni instructed the chaperones to wait. If they had indeed arrived at the academy, as Joni hoped, they would be greeted by the staff at any moment. The problem of the silent bus driver could be addressed at the appropriate time.

Increasingly, however, it seemed that this was not the case, and that no one was coming to greet them.

Joni gripped the back of her seat and stood, feeling her way to the open door. She called into the darkness:

"Hello?"

She heard nothing other than the popping and pinging of the coach's cooling engine, and the flutter of a passing bird's wings.

She turned to the young passengers in her care. She sensed their exhaustion and their anxiety. A long trip, now with an uncertain end. Some of the children in back were crying.

Joni called a chaperone meeting at the front. Amid frantic whispering, no one knew what to do.

"Out of range," explained Joni's cell phone, in an annoyingly patient voice.

One of them felt along the large dashboard for the operator's radio but could not locate the handset. He did notice that the driver's seat of cushioned plastic was still exceedingly warm.

Another chaperone, a brash nineteen-year-old named Joel, finally unfolded his cane and picked his way down the bus steps to the ground.

"It's a grassy field," he reported back. Then he yelled, to the driver or to anyone else who might be within earshot: "Hello! Is anybody there?"

"This is so wrong," said Joni, who, as the lead chaperone, felt as helpless as the little ones in her care. "I just can't understand it."

"Wait," said Joel, talking over her. "Do you hear that?"

They were all quiet, listening.

"Yes," said another.

Joni heard nothing aside from an owl hooting in the distance. "What?"

"I don't know. A . . . a humming."

"What? Mechanical?"

"Maybe. I don't know. It's more like . . . almost like a mantra from yoga class. You know, one of those sacred syllables?"

She listened longer. "I don't hear a thing, but . . . okay. Look, we have two choices. Close the door and stay here, and be helpless—or get everybody outside and mobilize them to find help."

No one wanted to stay. They had been on the bus too long.

"What if this is some test?" speculated Joel. "You know, part of the weekend."

Another murmured her agreement.

That sparked something in Joni. "Fine," she said. "If this is a test, then we're going to ace it."

They unloaded the children by rows, and shepherded them into tight columns where they could walk with one hand resting on the shoulder of the child in front of them. Some of the children acknowledged the "hum," responding to it, trying to replicate the noise for the others. Its presence seemed to calm them. Its source gave them all a destination.

Three chaperones led the way, sweeping their sticks over the surface of the field. The ground was rugged but largely clear of rocks or other treacherous obstacles.

Soon, they heard animal noises in the distance. Someone guessed donkeys, but most agreed no. It sounded like pigs.

A farm? Maybe the humming was a large generator? Some sort of feed machine grinding at night?

Their pace quickened until they reached an impediment: a low wooden rail fence. Two of the three leaders split up left and right, searching for an opening. One was located, and the group was herded to it, moving inside. The grass turned to dirt beneath their shoes, and the pig noises grew louder, nearer. They were on some sort of broad path, and the chaperones drew the children into tighter columns, striding forward until they reached a building of some sort. The path led directly to a large, open doorway, and they entered, calling out but receiving no answer.

They were inside a vast room of various contrapuntal noises. The hogs reacted to their presence with squeals of curiosity that frightened the children. They butted their tight pens and scraped their hooves against the straw-laden floor. Joni felt for the stalls lining either side of the group. The smell was of animal excrement, but also . . . something more foul. Something like charnel.

They had found the inside of the swine wing of a slaughterhouse, though none of them would have called it by that name.

The hum had become a voice for some of them. Those children felt compelled to break ranks, apparently responding to something familiar in the voice—and the chaperones had to round them up again, some by force. They initiated a new head count to make sure they were all still together.

While she was participating in the count, Joni finally heard the voice. She recognized it as her own, the strangest sensation—the voice seeming to originate inside her own head, hailing her, as in a dream.

They followed the call of the voice, walking forward down a wide ramp to a common area thick with the smell of charnel.

"Hello?" said Joni, her voice trembling—still hoping that the corny bus driver would answer them. "Can you help us?"

A being awaited them. A shadow akin to an eclipse. They felt its heat and sensed its immensity. The droning noise swelled, filled their heads beyond distraction, blanketing their most profound remaining sense—aural recognition—and leaving them in a state of near-suspended animation.

None of them heard the tender crinkling of the Master's burned flesh as he moved.

FALL 1944

THE OX-DRIVEN CART BUMPED OVER DIRT AND matted grass, rolling stubbornly through the countryside. The oxen were agreeable beasts, as are most castrated draught animals, their thin, braided tails swaying in sync like pendulum rods.

The driver's hands were leathered where he gripped the driving rope. The man seated next to the driver, his passenger, wore a long black gown over black pants. Around his neck hung the long holy beads of a Polish priest.

Yet this young man dressed in holy vestments was not a priest. He was not even Catholic.

He was a Jew in disguise.

An automobile approached from behind. It drew even with them on the rutted road, a military vehicle transporting Russian soldiers, then passed them on the left. The driver did not wave or even turn his head in acknowledgment, using his long stick to prod the slowed oxen as they pushed through the smoky exhaust of the diesel engine. "Doesn't matter how fast you travel," he said, once the fumes cleared. "In the end we all arrive at the same destination, eh, Father?"

Abraham Setrakian did not answer. Because he wasn't certain anymore that what the man said was true.

The thick bandage Setrakian wore around his neck was a ruse. He had learned to understand much of the Polish language, but he could not speak it well enough to pass.

"They beat you, Father," said the oxcart driver. "Broke your hands."

Setrakian regarded his young, mangled hands. The smashed knuckles had healed improperly during his time on the run. A local surgeon took pity on him and re-broke and reset the middle joints, which relieved some of the bone-on-bone grinding. He had some mobility in them now, more so than he might have hoped. The surgeon told him his joints would get progressively worse as he aged. Setrakian flexed them throughout the day, up to and then well past the point of pain, in an effort to increase their flexibility. The war cast a dark shadow over any man's hope for a long and productive life, but Setrakian had decided that, however much time he had left, he would never be considered a cripple.

He did not recognize this part of the country-side upon his return—but then how would he? He had arrived to this locale inside a closed, win-dowless train. He had never left camp until the uprising, and then—on the run, deep into the woods. He looked now for the train tracks, but, apparently, they had been pulled up. The train's path remained, however, its telltale scar running through the farmland. One year's time was not long enough for nature to reclaim that trail of infamy.

Setrakian climbed down off the cart near the final turn, with a blessing for the peasant driver. "Do not stay here long, Father," said the driver, before whipping his oxen into action. "There's a pall over this place."

Setrakian watched his beasts amble off, then walked up the beaten path. He came to a modest brick farmhouse set alongside an overgrown field tended to by a few workers. The extermination camp known as Treblinka was constructed to be impermanent. It was conceived as a temporary human slaughterhouse, constructed for maximum efficiency and intended to disappear completely once its purpose had been served. No tattooed arms as at Auschwitz; very little paperwork whatsoever. The camp was disguised as a train station complete with a false ticket window, a false station name ("Obermajdan"), and a fictitious list of connecting stations. The architects of the Operation Reinhard death camps had planned the perfect crime on a genocidal scale.

Soon after the prisoner uprising, Treblinka was indeed dismantled, torn down in the fall of 1943. The land was ploughed over, and a farm was erected on the site, with the intention of discouraging locals from trespassing and scavenging. The farmhouse was constructed using bricks recovered from the old gas chambers, and a former Ukrainian guard named Strebel and his family were installed as its occupants. The Ukrainian camp workers were former Soviet prisoners of war conscripted into service. The work of the camp—mass murder—affected one and all. Setrakian had seen for himself how these former prisoners themselves—especially the Ukrainians of German extraction, who were given greater responsibilities, such as commanding platoons or squads—succumbed to the corruption of the death camp and its opportunities for sadism as well as personal enrichment.

This man, Strebel, Setrakian could not conjure his face by name alone, but he remembered well the Ukrainians' black uniforms, as well as their carbines—and their cruelty. Word had reached Setrakian that Strebel and his family had only recently abandoned this farmland, fleeing ahead of the advancing Red Army. But Setrakian, in his position as country priest some sixty miles away, also was privy to tales describing a plague of evil that had settled over the region surrounding the former death camp. It was whispered that the Strebel family had disappeared one night without a word, without taking any possessions with them.

It was this last tale that intrigued Setrakian the most.

He had come to suspect he had gone at least partly, if not fully, insane inside the death camp. Had he seen what he thought he'd seen? Or was this great vampire feasting on Jewish prisoners some figment of his imagination, a coping mechanism, a golem to stand for the Nazi atrocities his mind could not bear to accept?

Only now did he feel strong enough to seek an answer. He went out past the brick house, walking among the workers tilling the field—only to discover that they were not laborers at all, but locals bearing digging tools from home, turning over soil in search of Jewish gold and jewelry lost in the massacre. Yet all they kept unearthing were barbed wire and the occasional chunk of bone.

They looked upon him with suspicion, as though there was a distinct code of conduct for looters, never mind vaguely defined areas of claim. Even his vestments did not slow their digging or melt their resolve. A few may have slowed and looked down—not in shame exactly, but in the manner of those who know better—and then waited for him to continue on before resuming their grave-robbing.

Setrakian walked on from the old camp site, leaving its outline and retracing his old escape route into the forest. After many wrong turns, he arrived at the old Roman ruin, which looked unchanged to his eye. He entered the cave where he had faced and destroyed the Nazi Zimmer, broken hands and all—hauling the being into the light of day and watching it cook in the sun.

As he looked around inside, he realized something. The scores on the floor, the worn path inside the entrance: the cave showed signs of recent habitation.

Setrakian exited quickly and felt his chest constrict as he stood outside the foul ruin. He did sense evil in the area. The sun was dipping low in the west, darkness soon to take the region.

Setrakian closed his eyes in the manner of a priest in prayer. But he was not appealing to a higher being. He was centering himself, pushing down his fear and accepting the task that had presented itself to him.

By the time he had returned to the farmhouse, the locals had all gone home, the fields as still and gray as the graveyard they were.

Setrakian entered the farmhouse. He poked about a bit, just enough to make sure that he was indeed alone there. In the parlor, he received a fright. On the small reading table next to the best chair in the room, a finely carved wooden smoking pipe lay on its side. Setrakian reached for the pipe, taking it into his crooked fingers—and knew instantly.

The handiwork was indeed his. He had crafted four of these, carved at the order of a Ukrainian captain at Christmastime 1942, to be given away as gifts.

The pipe trembled in Setrakian's hand as he imagined the guard Strebel sitting in this very room with his family, surrounded by the bricks of the death house, enjoying his tobacco and the fine ribbon of smoke trailing toward the ceiling—on the very site where the fire pits roared and the stench of human immolation rose like screams to the unhearing heavens.

Setrakian broke the pipe in his hands, snapping it in two, then dropping it to the floor and further crushing it with his heel, shivering with a fury he had not experienced in many months.

And then, as suddenly as it came—the mania passed. He was calm again.

He returned to the modest kitchen. He lit a single candle and placed it in the window facing the woods. And then he sat at the table.

Alone in the home, flexing his broken hands while he waited, he recalled the day he came upon the village church. He went seeking food, a man on the run, and discovered the religious house empty. All the Catholic priests had been rounded up and taken away. Setrakian discovered warm vestments in the small rectory adjacent to the church, and more out of necessity than any sort of plan—his clothes were tattered beyond repair, marking him as a refugee of some stripe, and the nights were very cold—he pulled them on. He came upon the ruse of the bandage, which no one questioned in a time of war. Even in silence, and perhaps out of a hunger for religion in that dark year, the villagers took to him, airing their confessions to this young man in holy garb who could only offer them a blessing with his mangled hands.

Setrakian was not the rabbi his family had intended him to become. He was something much different, and yet so oddly similar.

It was there, in that abandoned church, that he wrestled with what he had seen, at times wondering how any of it—from the sadism of the Nazis to the grotesquery of the great Vampire—could have been real. He had only his broken hands as proof. By then, the camp, as he had been told by other refugees to whom he offered "his" church as sanctuary—peasants on the run from the Armia Krajowa, deserters from the Wehrmacht or the Gestapo—had been wiped off the face of the earth.

After dusk, when full night had claimed the countryside, an eerie silence settled over the farm. The countryside is anything but quiet at night, and yet the zone surrounding the former death camp was hushed and solemn. It was as though the night were holding its breath.

A visitor arrived soon enough. He appeared in the window, his worm-white face illuminated by the candle flame flickering against the thin, imperfect glass. Setrakian had left the door unlocked, and the visitor walked inside, moving stiffly as though recovering from some great, debilitating disease.

Setrakian turned to face the man with trembling disbelief. SS-Sturmscharführer Hauptmann, his former taskmaster inside the camp. The man responsible for the carpentry shop, and all of the so-called "court Jews" who supplied skilled personal services to the SS and the Ukrainian staff. His familiar, all-black Schutzstaffel uniform—always pristine—was now in tatters, the hanging shreds revealing twin SS tattoos on his now-hairless forearms. His polished buttons were missing, as were his belt and black cap. The death-head insignia of the SS-Totenkopfverbände remained on his worn black collar. His black leather boots, always buffed to a high sheen, were now cracked and caked with grime. His hands, mouth, and neck were stained with the dried black blood of former victims, and a halo of flies clouded the air around his head.

He carried burlap sacks in his long hands. For what reason, wondered Setrakian, had this former ranking officer of the Schutzstaffel come to collect earth from the site of the former Treblinka camp? This loam fertilized with the gas and ash of genocide?

The vampire looked down upon him with rusty red eyes, its gaze remote.

Abraham Setrakian.

The voice came from somewhere, not the vampire's mouth. Its bloodied lips never moved.

You escaped the pit.

The voice within Setrakian was deep and broad, reverberating in him as though his spine were a tuning fork. That same, many-tongued voice.

The great vampire. The very one he had encountered inside the camp—speaking through Hauptmann.

"Sardu," said Setrakian, addressing him by the name of the human form he had taken, the noble giant of legend, Jusef Sardu.

I see you are dressed as a holy man. You once spoke of your God. Do you believe He delivered you from the burning pit?

Setrakian said, "No."

Do you still wish to destroy me?

Setrakian did not speak. But the answer was yes.

It seemed to read his thought, its voice burbling with what could only be described as pleasure.

You are resilient, Abraham Setrakian. Like the leaf that refuses to fall.

"What is this now? Why are you still here?"

You mean Hauptmann. He was made to facilitate my involvement in the camp. In the end, I turned him. And he then fed upon the young officers he once favored. He had a taste for pure Aryan blood.

"Then—there are others."

The chief administrator. And the camp doctor.

Eichhorst, thought Setrakian. And Dr. Dreverhaven. Yes indeed. Setrakian remembered them both well.

"And Strebel and his family?"

Strebel interested me not at all, except as a meal. Those bodies we destroy after feeding, before they begin to turn. You see, food here has become scarce. Your war is a nuisance. Why create more mouths to feed?

"Then—what do you want here?"

Hauptmann's head tilted unnaturally, his full throat clucking once, like a frog's.

Why don't we call it nostalgia. I miss the efficiencies of the camp. I have become spoiled by the convenience of a human buffet. And now—I am tired of answering your questions.

"One more then." Setrakian looked again at the sacks of soil in Hauptmann's hands. "One month before the uprising, Hauptmann directed me to construct a very large cabinet. He even supplied the wood, a very thick ebony grain, imported. I was given a drawing to copy, carving into the top doors."

Indeed. You do good work, Jew.

A "special project," Hauptmann had called it. At the time, Setrakian, having no choice in the matter, feared he was building furniture for an SS officer in Berlin. Perhaps even Hitler himself.

But no. It was much worse.

History told me the camp would not last. None of the great experiments do. I knew that the feast would end, and that I would be moving soon. One of the Allies' bombs had struck an unintended target: my bed. So I needed a new one. Now I am sure to keep it with me at all times.

Setrakian's anger, not fear, was the cause of his shaking.

He had built the great vampire's coffin.

And now, Hauptmann must feed. I am not at all surprised that you returned here, Abraham Setrakian. It seems we are both sentimental about this place.

Hauptmann dropped his bags of dirt. Setrakian stood as the vampire started toward the table, backing up against the wall.

Do not worry, Abraham Setrakian. I will not give you to the animals after. I think you should join us. Your character is strong. Your bones will heal, and your hands will again serve us.

Up close, Setrakian felt Hauptmann's uncanny heat. The vampire radiated its fever, and stunk of the earth it had been collecting. Its lipless mouth parted and Setrakian could see the tip of the stinger inside, ready to strike at him.

He looked into vampire Hauptmann's red eyes, and hoped that the Sardu Thing was indeed looking back.

Hauptmann's dirty hand closed around the bandage covering Setrakian's neck. The vampire pulled the gauze away, and in doing so uncovered a bright silver throat piece covering the esophagus and major arteries. Hauptmann's eyes widened as it stumbled backward, repelled by the protective silver plate Setrakian had hired his village smith to fashion.

Hauptmann felt the opposite wall at his back. He groaned, weakened and confused. But Setrakian could see that he was only readying his next attack.

Resilient to the end.

As Hauptmann ran at Setrakian, Setrakian produced, from the folds of his robe, a silver crucifix whose long end had been sharpened to a point, and met him halfway.

The slaying of the Nazi vampire was, in the end, an act of pure release. For Setrakian, it represented an opportunity for revenge upon Treblinka soil, as well as a blow against the great vampire and his mysterious ways. But, more than any of that, it served as confirmation of Setrakian's sanity.

Yes, he had seen what he had seen in the camp.

Yes, the myth was true.

And yes, the truth was terrible.

The slaying sealed Setrakian's fate. He thenceforth dedicated his life to educating himself about the *strigoi*—and hunting them down.

He shed his priestly vestments that night, trading them for the garments of a simple farmer, and burned clean the whitish tip of his crucifixion dagger. On his way out, he overturned the candle onto his robe and some rags, and walked off with the light from the flames of the cursed farmhouse flashing against his back.

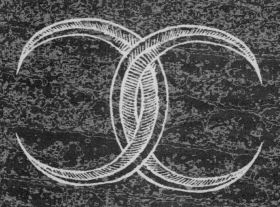

Knickerbocker Loans and Curios, East 118th Street, Spanish Harlem

Setrakian unlocked the pawnshop door and raised the security gate, and Fet, waiting outside like a customer, imagined the old man repeating this routine every day for the past thirty-five years. The shop-owner came out into the sunlight, and for just a moment everything might have been normal. An old man squinting into the sun on a street in New York City. The moment inspired nostalgia in Fet, rather than encouragement. It did not seem to him that there were many more "normal" moments left.

Setrakian, in a tweed vest without jacket, white shirtsleeves rolled just past his wrists, looked at the large van. The door and side wall read: MANHATTAN DEPARTMENT OF PUBLIC WORKS.

Fet told him, "I borrowed it."

The old professor appeared pleased and intrigued. "I wonder, can you get another?"

"Why? Where are we going?"

"We cannot remain here any longer."

Eph sat down on the flat exercise mat inside the odd-angled storage room on the top floor of Setrakian's home. Zack sat there with one leg bent, his knee as high as his cheek, arms hugging his thigh. Zack looked ragged, like a boy sent off to sleepaway camp who came back changed, and not for the better. Silver-backed mirrors surrounded them, giving Eph the feeling of being watched by many old eyes. The window frame within the iron bars had been hastily boarded over, a bandage uglier than the wound it covered.

Eph studied his son's face, trying to read it. He was worried about the boy's sanity, as he was worried about his own. He rubbed his mouth in preparation for talking, and felt roughness around the edges of his lips and chin, realizing he hadn't shaved in days.

"I checked the parenting handbook earlier," he began. "Unfortunately there was no chapter about vampires."

He tried to smile, but wasn't sure it worked. He wasn't sure his smile was persuasive anymore. He wasn't sure anyone should be smiling now.

"Okay, so, this is going to sound twisted—and it *is* twisted. But let me get it out. You know your mom loved you, Z. More even than you know, as much as a mother can love a son. That's why she and I went through all we did, what felt to you at times like a tug-of-war—because neither one of us could bear being apart from you. Because you're it. I know that children sometimes blame themselves for their parents' breakup. But you were the one thing holding us together. And driving us crazy fighting over you."

"Dad, you don't have to—"

"I know, I know. Cut to it, right? But no. This stuff you need to hear, and right now. Maybe I need to hear it too, okay? We need to set each other straight. Put it right out in front of us. A mother's love is . . . it's like a force. It's beyond simple human affection. It's soul-deep. A father's love—my love for you, Z—it's the strongest thing in my life, absolutely it is. But this thing has made me realize that there's something about maternal love—it might just be the strongest human spiritual bond there is."

He checked to see how this was going with Zack. Couldn't tell.

"And now this thing, this plague, this awful . . . it's taken who she was and burned off all that was good in her. All that was right and true. All that was, as we understand it, human. Your mom . . . she was beautiful, she was caring, she was . . . she was also crazy, in the way all devoted mothers are. But you were her great gift to the world. That's how she saw you. That's what you are still. That part of her lives on. But now—she is not herself anymore. She is not Kelly Goodweather, not Mom—and this is hard for both of us to accept. All that remains of what she was, as far as I can tell, is her bond with you. Because that bond is sacred, and it never dies. What we call love, in our sappy greeting-card way, is evidently something much deeper than we humans imagined. Her human love for you has . . . it seems to have shifted, has morphed, into this kind of want, this need. Where she is now, this bad place? She wants you there with her. It's not bad to her, or evil, or dangerous. She just wants you with her. And what you need to know is that this is all because your mother loved you so completely."

Zack nodded. He couldn't or wouldn't speak.

"Now, that said, we have to keep you safe from her. She looks different now, right? That's because she *is* different—fundamentally different—and it's not easy to face that. I can't make this right for you except to protect you from her. From what she has become. That's my new job now, as your parent, as your father. If you think of your mom, as she originally was, and what she would do to save you from any threat to your health, to your safety . . . well, you tell me. What would she do?"

Zack nodded, answering immediately. "She would hide me."

"She would take you away. Remove you from the threat, get you to a safe place." Eph listened to what he was saying. "Just pick you up and . . . run. I'm right, aren't I?"

"You're right," said Zack.

"Okay, so—being the overprotective mom? That's my job now."

Brooklyn

ERIC JACKSON PHOTOGRAPHED the window burn from three different angles. He always carried a small Canon digital camera when he was on duty, along with his gun and his badge.

Acid etching was the thing now. Craft-store etching product usually mixed with shoe polish, marking on glass or Plexiglas. It didn't show up immediately, burning into the glass in the space of hours. The longer the acid-etched tag remained, the more permanent it became.

He stood back to size up the shape. Six black appendages radiating from a red center mass. He clicked back through his camera memory. Another one, taken yesterday in Bay Ridge, only not as well-defined. And another, in Canarsie, looking more like an oversized asterisk but evincing the same tight lines.

Jackson knew Phade's work anywhere. True, this wasn't like his usual throw-ups—this was amateur work compared to that—but the fine arcs and perfect free-hand proportion were unmistakable.

Dude was going all-city, sometimes in one night. How was that possible?

Eric Jackson was a member of the New York Police Department's Citywide Vandals Taskforce, his job to track and prevent vandalism. He believed in the gospel of the NYPD as it pertained to graffiti. Even the most beautifully colored and detailed graffiti throw-up represented an affront to public order. An invitation to others to consider the urban environment theirs to do with as they pleased. Freedom of expression was always the miscreant's way out, but littering was an act of expression also, and you still got nicked for it. Order was a fragile thing, with chaos always just a few steps away.

The city was seeing that now, firsthand.

Riots had claimed whole blocks in the South Bronx. Nighttime was the worst. Jackson kept waiting for a call from a captain that would put him back in the old uniform and out on the street. But no word yet. Not a lot of radio chatter at all, whenever he switched it on inside his car. So he kept on doing what he was paid to do.

The governor had resisted calls for the National Guard, but he was just a guy in Albany, weighing his political future. Supposedly, with so many units still in Iraq and Afghanistan, the guard was undermanned and underequipped—but, looking at the black smoke in the distant sky, Jackson would have welcomed any help.

Jackson dealt with vandals in all five boroughs, but nobody bombed as much of the city's façade as Phade. Dude was everywhere. Must have slept all day, tagged all night. He was fifteen or sixteen now, had been getting up since he was twelve. That was the age most taggers start, toying up at schools, on newspaper boxes, etc. In surveillance photos, Phade's face was always obscured, usually by a Yankees cap tucked underneath a sweatshirt hood, sometimes even an aerosol mask. He wore typical tagger get-up: cargo pants with many pockets, a backpack for his Krylons, hi-top kicks.

Most vandals work in tagging crews, but not Phade. He was a young legend, moving with apparent impunity throughout diverse neighborhoods. He was said to carry a stolen set of transit keys, including a skeleton that unlocked subway cars. His tags earned respect. The typical profile of a young tagger is low self-esteem, a desire for peer recognition, a distorted view of fame. Phade fit none of these traits. His signature wasn't a tag—usually a nickname or a repetitive motif—but his style itself. His pieces jumped off walls. Jackson's own suspicion—long since moved from a hunch to a foregone certainty—was that Phade was likely obsessive-compulsive, perhaps showing symptoms of Asperger's syndrome or even full-spectrum autism.

Jackson understood this, in part, because he was an obsessive himself. He carried a full book on Phade, quite similar in appearance to the "piece books" taggers carried, featuring their graffiti outlines in a black-cover Cachet sketchbook. As one of five officers assigned to the GHOST unit within the Vandals Taskforce—the Graffiti Habitual Offender Suppression Team—he was responsible for maintaining a graffiti offender databank cross-referencing tags and throw-ups with addresses. People who consider graffiti a kind of "street art" think of brightly colored, Wild Style bubble bombs on building murals and subway cars. They don't think of tagging crews etching storefronts, competing for high-profile—and often dangerous—"gets." Or, more often, marking gang territory, establishing name recognition and intimidation.

The other four GHOST cops had stopped showing up for shifts. Some radio reports had NYPD officers deserting the city like the New Orleans cops after Hurricane Katrina, but Jackson couldn't believe that. Something else was happening—something beyond this sickness spreading throughout the boroughs. You're sick, you bang in. You get your shift covered so you don't leave a brother to pick up your slack. These claims of abandonment and cowardice offended him like some incompetent tagger's clumsy-ass signature over a freshly painted wall. Jackson would believe this crazy vampire shit people were talking before he'd accept that his guys had turned tail and skedaddled to Jersey.

He got inside his unmarked car and drove down the quiet street to Coney Island. He did this three days a week, at least. It was his favorite spot growing up, but his parents didn't take him there nearly as much as he'd have liked. While he'd abandoned his pledge to go every day when he was a grown-up, he went often enough for lunch to make it okay.

The boardwalk was empty, as he had expected. The autumn day was certainly warm enough, but with the mad flu, amusement was the last thing on people's minds. He hit Nathan's Famous and found the place deserted but not locked up. Abandoned. He had worked at this very hot-dog stand after high school, so he went back behind the counter and into the kitchen. He shooed away two rats, then wiped down the cooking surface. The fridge was still cold inside, so he pulled out two beef dogs. He found the buns and a cellophane-covered tin of red onions. He liked onions, especially the way the vandals winced when he got up in their face after lunch.

The dogs cooked fast, and he stepped outside to eat. The Cyclone and the Wonder Wheel were still and quiet, seagulls perched on the uppermost railings. Another seagull flew close, then darted away from the top of the wheel at the last moment. Jackson looked closer and realized that the critters sitting atop the structure weren't birds at all.

They were rats. Lots of rats, dotting the top edges of the structure. Trying to grab birds. What in the hell?

He continued down the boardwalk, passing Shoot the Freak, one of Coney Island's landmark attractions. From a railed promontory, he looked down into the alley-like shooting gallery cluttered with fencing, spattered barrels, and assorted mannequin heads and bowling pins set upon rusted racks for target practice. Along the railing were six paintball guns chained to a table. The sign listed the prices, promising a LIVE HUMAN TARGET.

The brick side walls were decorated with graffiti, creating more character. But among the fake white Krylon tags and weak bubble throw-ups, Jackson noticed another of Phade's designs. Another six-limbed figure, this one in black and orange. And, near it, in the same colors, a design of lines and dots similar to the code he had been seeing all over town.

Then he saw the freak. The freak was dressed in heavy black armor, like riot gear, covering his entire body. A helmet and mask with protective goggles hid his face. The orange-painted shield he normally carried in order to deflect paintball projectiles stood against a low section of chain-link fence.

The freak stood at the far corner of the shooting alley, a can of spray paint in its gloved hand, marking up the wall.

"Hey!" Jackson called down to him.

The freak didn't acknowledge him. It kept right on tagging.

"Hey!" called Jackson, louder now. "NYPD! I wanna talk to you!"

Still no response or reaction.

Jackson picked up each of the carbine-like paintball guns, hoping for a free shot. He found one with a handful of orange balls still inside its opaque plastic feeder. He shouldered the weapon and fired low, the carbine kicking and the paintball exploding in the dirt at the freak's boot.

The freak didn't flinch. It finished its tag and then dropped the empty can and started toward the underside of the railing where Jackson stood.

"Hey, asshole, I said I wanna talk to you."

The freak did not stop. Jackson unloaded three blasts at its chest, exploding red. Then the freak passed below Jackson's angle of fire, heading underneath him.

Jackson went to the railing, lifting himself over it and dangling a moment before dropping down. From there, he had a better view of the freak's handiwork.

It was Phade. No doubt in Jackson's mind. His pulse quickened and he started for the only door.

Inside was a tiny changing room, the floor spattered with paint. Beyond was a narrow hallway, and along it he saw, discarded, the freak's helmet, gloves, goggles, body armor overalls, and other gear. Jackson realized then what he had only previously begun to understand: Phade wasn't just an opportunist using the riots as cover to blanket the city with his tags. No—Phade was linked to the unrest somehow. His markings, his throw-ups: he was part of this.

At the end, he turned into a small office with a counter and a phone, stacks of paintball loads in egg cartons, and broken carbines.

On the swivel chair was an open backpack stuffed with Krylon cans and loose markers. Phade's gear.

Then a noise behind him and he whipped around. There was the tagger, shorter than Jackson had imagined, wearing a paint-stained hoodie, a silver-on-black Yankees cap, and an aerosol mask.

"Hey," said Jackson, all he could think to say at first. It had been such a long hunt, he never expected to find his man so abruptly. "I wanna talk to you."

Phade said nothing, staring, his eyes dark and low beneath the brim of his ball cap. Jackson moved to the side in case Phade was thinking of ditching his backpack and trying to make a run for it.

"You're a pretty slippery character," Jackson said. Jackson had his camera in his jacket pocket, ready as ever. "First of all, take off the face mask and hat. I want you to smile for the birdie."

Phade moved slowly—not at all, at first, but then its paint-spattered hands came up, pulling back its hood, removing its cap, and pulling down its aerosol mask.

The camera remained at Jackson's eye, but he never pushed the button. What he saw through the lens surprised him at first—then transfixed him.

This wasn't Phade at all. Couldn't be. This was a Puerto Rican girl.

She had red paint around her mouth, as though she had been huffing it, getting high. But no: huffed paint leaves an even, thin coat around the mouth. These were thick drops of red, some of it dried below her chin. Her chin dropped then, and the stinger lashed out, the vampire artist leaping onto Jackson's chest and shoulders and driving him back against the counter, drinking him dry.

The Flatlands

FLATLANDS WAS A neighborhood near the southern shore of Brooklyn between Canarsie and the coastal Marine Park. As with most New York City neighborhoods, it had undergone many significant demographical changes throughout the twentieth century. The library currently offered French-Creole books for Haitian residents and immigrants from other Caribbean nations, as well as reading programs in coordination with local yeshivas for children from Orthodox Jewish families.

Fet's shop was a small storefront in a strip mall around the corner from Flatlands Avenue. No electricity, but Fet's old telephone still gave out a dial tone. The front of the store was used mostly for storage, and not designed to service walk-in customers; in fact, the rat sign over the door was specifically meant to discourage window shoppers. His workshop and garage were in back; that was where they loaded in the most essential items from Setrakian's basement armory—books, weapons, and other wares.

The similarity between Setrakian's basement armory and Fet's workshop was not lost on Eph. Fet's enemies were rodents and insects, and, for that reason, the space was filled with cages, telescoping syringe poles, black-light wands, and miners' helmets for night hunting. Snake tongs, animal control poles, odor eliminators, dart guns, even throw nets. Powders, trapping gloves, and a lab area over a small sink, with some rudimentary veterinary equipment for taking blood or sampling captured prey.

The only curious feature was a deep stack of *Real Estate* magazines lying around a gnarly La-Z-Boy recliner. Where others might keep a stash of porn tucked away in their workshop, Fet had these. "I like the pictures," he said. "The houses with their warm lights on, against the blue dusk. So beautiful. I like to try to imagine the lives of people who might live inside such a place. Happy people."

Nora entered, taking a break from unloading, drinking from a bottle of water, one hand on her hip. Fet handed Eph a heavy key ring.

"Three locks for the front door, three for the back." He demonstrated, showing the order of the keys as they were organized along the ring. "These open the cabinets—left to right."

"Where are you off to?" asked Eph, as Fet headed for the door.

"Old man's got something for me to do."

Nora said, "Pick us up some takeout on your way back."

"Those were the days," said Fet, moving out to the second van.

Setrakian brought Fet the item he had carried in his lap from Manhattan. A small bundle of rags, with something wrapped inside. He handed it to Fet.

"You will return underground," said Setrakian. "Find those ducts that connect to the mainland, and close them."

Fet nodded, the old man's request as good as an order. "Why alone?"

"You know those tunnels better than anyone else. And Zachary needs time with his father."

Fet nodded. "How is the kid?"

Setrakian sighed. "For him, there is first the abject horror of the circumstances, the terror of this new reality. And then there is the *Unheimlich*. The uncanny. I speak here of the mother. The familiar and the foreign together, and the feeling of anxiety it inspires. Drawing him, and yet repulsing him."

"You might as well be talking about the doc, too."

"Indeed. Now, about this task—you must be swift." He pointed to the package. "The timer will give you three minutes. Only three."

Fet peeked inside the oil-stained rags: three sticks of dynamite and a small mechanical timer. "Jesus—it looks like an egg timer."

"So it is. 1950s analog. Analog avoids mistakes, you see. Crank it all the way to the right, and then run. The small box underneath will generate the necessary spark to detonate the sticks. Three minutes. A soft-boiled egg. Do you think you can find a place to hide that fast down there?"

Fet nodded. "I don't see why not. How long ago did you assemble this?"

"Some time ago," said Setrakian. "It will still work."

"You had this around—in your basement?"

"Volatile weapons I kept in the back of the cellar. A small vault, sealed, concrete wall and asbestos. Hidden from city inspectors. Or nosy exterminators."

Fet nodded, carefully wrapping up the explosive and tucking the package underneath his arm. He moved closer to Setrakian, speaking privately. "Level with me here, professor. I mean, what are we doing? Unless I'm missing something—I don't see any way to stop this. Slow it down, sure. But destroying them one by one—that's like trying to kill every rat in the city by hand. It's spreading too fast."

"That much is true," said Setrakian. "We need a way to destroy more efficiently. But, by that same token, I do not believe the Master to be satisfied with exponential exposure."

Fet digested the big words, then nodded. "Because hot diseases burn out. That's what the doc said. They run out of hosts."

"Indeed," Setrakian said, with a tired expression. "There is a greater plan at work. What it is—I hope we never have to find out."

"Whatever it is," said Fet, patting the rags beneath his arm, "count on me to be right at your side."

Setrakian watched Fet climb into the van and drive off. He liked the Russian, even if he suspected that the exterminator enjoyed the killing only too much. There are men who bloom in chaos. You call them heroes or villains, depending on which side wins the war, but until the battle call they are but normal men who long for action, who lust for the opportunity to throw off the routine of their normal lives like a cocoon and come into their own. They sense a destiny larger than themselves, but only when structures collapse around them do these men become warriors.

Fet was one of them. Unlike Ephraim, Fet had no question about his calling or his deeds. Not that he was stupid or uncaring—quite the contrary. He had a sharp, instinctive intelligence and was a natural tactician. And once set on a course, he never faltered, never stopped.

A great ally to have at one's side for the Master's final call.

Setrakian returned inside, pulling open a small crate full of yellowing newspaper. From inside he delicately retrieved some chemistry glassware—more alchemist's kitchen than science lab. Zack was nearby, chewing on the last of their granola bars. He found a silver sword and hefted it, handling the weapon with appropriate care, finding it surprisingly heavy. Then he touched the crumbling hem of a chest plate made of thick animal hide, horsehair, and sap.

"Fourteenth century," Setrakian told him. "Dating from the beginning of the Ottoman Empire, and the era of the Black Plague. You see the neckpiece?" He pointed out the high front shield rising to the wearer's chin. "From a hunter in the fourteenth century, his name lost to history. A museum piece, of no modern use to us. But I couldn't leave it behind."

"Seven centuries ago?" said Zack, his fingertips running along the brittle shell. "That old? If they've been around for so long, and if they have so much power, then why did they stay hidden?"

"Power revealed is power sacrificed," said Setrakian. "The truly powerful exert their influence in ways unseen, unfelt. Some would say that a thing visible is a thing vulnerable."

Zack examined the side of the chest plate, where a cross had been tanned into the hide. "Are they devils?"

Setrakian did not know how to answer that. "What do you think?"

"I guess it depends."

"On what?"

"On if you believe in God."

Setrakian nodded. "I think that is quite correct."

"Well?" said Zack. "Do you? Believe in God?"

Setrakian winced, then hoped the boy had not seen it. "An old man's beliefs matter little. I am the past. You, the future. What are your beliefs?"

Zack moved on to a handheld mirror backed in true silver. "My mom said God made us in His image. And He created everything."

Setrakian nodded, understanding the question implicit in the boy's response. "It is called a paradox. When two valid premises appear contradictory. Usually it means that one premise is faulty."

"But why would He make us so that . . . that we could turn into them?"

"You should ask Him."

The boy said quietly, "I have."

Setrakian nodded, patting the boy on the shoulder. "He never answered me either. Sometimes it is up to us to discover the answers for ourselves. And sometimes we never do."

An awkward situation, and yet Zack appealed to Setrakian. The boy had a bright curiosity and an earnestness that reflected well upon his generation.

"I am told boys your age like knives," Setrakian said, locating one and presenting it to the boy. A four-inch, folding silver blade with a brown bone grip.

"Wow." Zack worked the locking mechanism to close it, then opened it again. "I should probably check with my dad, make sure it's okay."

"I believe it fits perfectly in your pocket. Why don't you see?" He watched Zack collapse the blade and slide the grip into his pants pocket. "Good. Every boy should have a knife. Give it a name and it is yours forever."

"A name?" said Zack.

"One must always name a weapon. You cannot trust that which you cannot call by name."

Zack patted his pocket, his gaze faraway. "That's going to take some thinking."

Eph came over, noticing Zack and Setrakian together and sensing that something personal had passed between them.

Zack's hand went deep into his knife pocket, but he said nothing.

"There is a paper bag in the front seat of the van," said Setrakian. "It contains a sandwich. You must keep strong."

Zack said, "Not bologna again."

"My apologies," said Setrakian, "but it was on special the last time I went to market. This is the last of it. I put on some nice mustard. Also there are two good Drake's Cakes in the bag. You might enjoy one and then bring the other back for me."

Zack nodded, his father tousling his hair as he

went to the rear exit. "Lock the van doors when you get in there, okay?"

"I know . . ."

Eph watched him go, seeing him climb inside the passenger door of the van parked right outside. To Setrakian, Eph said, "You okay?"

"I am well enough. Here. I have something for you."

Eph received a lacquered wooden case. He opened the top, revealing a Glock in clean condition save for where the serial number had been filed off. Around it were five magazines of ammunition wedged into gray foam.

Eph said, "This would appear to be highly illegal."

"And highly useful. Those are silver bullets, mind you. Specially made."

Eph lifted the weapon out of the box, turning so that there was no chance of Zack seeing him. "I feel like the Lone Ranger."

"He had the right idea, didn't he? But what he didn't have was expanding tips. These bullets will fragment inside the body, burst. One shot anywhere in the trunk of a *strigoi* should do the trick."

The presentation had about it a hint of ceremony. Eph said, "Maybe Fet should have one."

"Vasiliy likes the nail gun. He is more manually inclined."

"And you like the sword."

"It is best to stay with what one is accustomed to, in times of trouble such as these." Nora came over, drawn by the strange sight of the gun. "I have another, medium-length silver dagger I think would suit you perfectly, Dr. Martinez."

She nodded, both hands in her pockets. "It's the only kind of jewelry I want just now."

Eph returned his weapon to the case, closing the top. This question was easier with Nora here. "What do you think happened up on that rooftop?" he asked Setrakian. "With the Master surviving the sun? Does it mean it is different from the rest?"

"Without doubt, it is different. It is their progenitor."

Nora said, "Right. Okay. And so we know—painfully well—how subsequent generations of vampires are created. Through stinger infection and such. But who created the first? And how?"

"Right," said Eph. "How can the chicken come before the egg?"

"Indeed," said Setrakian, pulling his wolf's-head-handled walking stick from the wall, leaning on it for support. "I believe the secret to all of this lies in the Master's making."

Nora said, "What secret?"

"The key to his undoing."

They were silent for a moment, absorbing this. Eph said, "Then—you know something."

Setrakian said, "I have a theory, which has been substantiated, at least in part, by what we witnessed on that rooftop. But I do not wish to be wrong, for it would sidetrack us, and as we all know, time is sand now and the hourglass is no longer being turned by human hands."

Nora said, "If sunlight didn't destroy it, then silver probably won't either."

"Its host body can be maimed and even killed," said Setrakian. "Ephraim succeeded in cutting it. But no, you are correct. We cannot assume that silver alone will be enough."

Eph said, "You've spoken of others. Seven Original Ancients, you said. The Master and six others, three Old World, three New World. Where are they in all this?"

"That is something I have been wondering about myself."

"Do we know, are they with him in this? I assume they are."

"On the contrary," said Setrakian. "Against him, wholeheartedly. Of that I am certain."

"And their creation? These beings came about at the same time, or in the same manner?"

"I can't imagine some other answer, yes."

Nora asked, "What does the lore say about the first vampires?"

"Very little, in fact. Some have tried to tie it to Judas, or the story of Lilith, but that is popular revisionist fiction. However . . . there is one book. One source."

Eph looked around. "Point me to the box. I'll get it."

"This is a book I do not yet possess. One book I have spent a fair portion of my life trying to acquire."

"Let me guess," said Eph. *The Vampire Hunter's Guide to Saving the World.*"

"Close. It is called the *Occido Lumen*. Strictly

translated, it means *I Kill the Light*, or, by extension, *The Fallen Light*." Setrakian produced the auction catalog from Sotheby's, opening it to a folded page.

The book was listed, although in the area where a picture should have run was a graphic reading NO IMAGE AVAILABLE.

"What is it about?" asked Eph.

"It is hard to explain. And even harder to accept. During my tenure in Vienna, I became, by necessity, fluent with many occult systems: Tarot, Qabbalah, Enochian Magick . . . everything and anything that helped me understand the fundamental questions I faced. They were all difficult subjects to fit in a curriculum but, for reasons I shall not divulge now, the university found abundant patronage for my research. It was during those years that I first heard of the *Lumen*. A bookseller from Leipzig came to me with a set of black-and-white photographs. Grainy stills of a few of the book's pages. His demands were outrageous. I had acquired quite a few *grimoires* from this seller—and for some of them he had commanded a handsome sum—but this . . . this was ridiculous. I did my research and found that, even among scholars, the book was considered a myth, a scam, a hoax. The literary equivalent of an urban legend. The volume was said to contain the exact nature and origin of all *strigoi* but, more important, it names all of the Seven Original Ancients . . . Three weeks later I traveled to the man's bookshop—a modest store in Nalewski Street. It was closed. I never heard from him again."

Nora said, "The seven names—they would include Sardu's?"

"Precisely," said Setrakian. "And to learn his name—his true name—would give us a hold on him."

"You're telling me that all we are looking for is the most expensive *White Pages* in the world?" said Eph.

Setrakian smiled gently and handed over the catalog to Eph. "I understand your skepticism. I do. To a modern man, a man of science—even one who has seen all that you have—ancient knowledge seems archaic. Creaky. A curiosity. But know this. Names do hold the essence of the thing. And, yes—even names listed in a directory. Names, letters, numbers, when known in depth, possess enormous power. Everything in our universe is ciphered and to know the cipher is to know the thing—and to know the thing is to command it. I once met a man, a very wise man, who could cause instant death by enunciating a six-syllable word. One word, Eph—but very few men know it. Now, imagine what that book contains . . ."

Nora read the catalog over Eph's shoulder. "And it's coming up for auction in two days?"

Setrakian said, "Something of an incredible coincidence, don't you think?"

Eph looked at him. "I doubt it."

"Correct. I believe this is all part of a puzzle. This book has a very dark and complicated provenance. When I tell you it is believed to be cursed, I don't mean that someone fell sick once after reading it. I mean that terrible occurrences surround its very appearance whenever it surfaces. Two auction houses that listed it previously burned to the ground before the bidding began. A third withdrew the item and closed its doors permanently. The item is now valued at between fifteen and twenty-five million dollars."

"Fifteen and twenty-five . . ." said Nora, puffing her cheeks. "This is a book we're talking about?"

"Not just any book." Setrakian took back the catalog. "We must acquire it. There is no other alternative."

Nora said, "Do they take personal checks?"

"That is the problem. At this price, there is very little chance we may procure it by legitimate means."

Eph darkened. "That's Eldritch Palmer money," he said.

"Precisely," said Setrakian, nodding ever so slightly. "And through him, Sardu—the Master."

Fet's Blog

BACK AGAIN. STILL trying to sort this thing out.

See, I think people's problem is, they're paralyzed by disbelief.

A vamp is some guy in a satin cape. Slicked-back hair, white makeup, funny accent. Two holes in the neck, and he turns into a bat, flies away.

I've seen that movie, right? Whatever.

Okay. Now look up Sacculina.

What the hell, you're already on the Internet anyway.

Go ahead. I did.

You back already? Good.

Now you know that Sacculina is a genus of parasitic barnacles that attack crabs.

And who cares, right? Why am I wasting your time?

What the female Sacculina does after her larva molts is she injects herself into the crab's body through a vulnerable joint in its armor. She gets in there and begins sprouting these root-like appendages that spread all throughout the crab's body, even around its eyestalks.

Now, once the crab's body is enslaved, the female then emerges as a sac. The male Sacculina joins her now, and guess what? Mating time.

Eggs incubate and mature inside the hostage crab, which is forced to devote all its energy to caring for this family of parasites that controls it.

The crab is a host. A drone. Utterly possessed by this different species, and compelled to care for the invader's eggs as if they were its own.

Who cares, right? Barnacles and crabs?

My point is: there are plenty of examples of this in nature.

Creatures invading bodies of species completely unlike their own and changing their essential function.

It's proven. It's known.

And yet we believe we're above all this. We're humans, right? Top of the food chain. We eat, we don't get eaten. We take, not get taken.

It's said that Copernicus (I can't be the only one who thought it was Galileo) took Earth out of the center of the universe.

And Darwin took humans out of the center of the living world.

So why do we still insist on believing we are somehow something more than animals?

Look at us. Essentially a collection of cells coordinated by chemical signals.

What if some invading organism seized control of these signals? Started to take us over, one by one. Rewriting our very nature, converting us to their own means?

Impossible, you say?

Why? You think the human race is "too big to fail"?

Okay. Now stop reading this. Stop cruising the Internet for answers and go out and grab yourself some silver and rise up against these things—before it is too late.

The Black Forest Solutions Facility

GABRIEL BOLIVAR, THE only remaining member of the original four "survivors" of Regis Air Flight 753, waited in a dirt-walled hollow deep beneath the drainage floor of Slaughterhouse #3, two stories below the Black Forest Solutions meatpacking facility.

The Master's oversize coffin lay atop a beam of rock and soil, in the absolute darkness of the underground chamber—and yet its heat signature was strong and distinct, the coffin glowing in Bolivar's vision, as though lit brightly from within. Enough so that Bolivar could perceive the detail of the carved edging near the double-hinged top doors.

Such was the intensity of the Master's ambient body temperature, radiating its glory.

Bolivar was well into the second stage of vampiric evolution. The pain of the transformation had all but receded, alleviated in large part by daily feedings, the red blood meal nourishing his body in a manner akin to protein and water building human muscle.

His new circulatory system was complete, his arteries now delivering sustenance to the chambers of his torso. His digestive system had become simplified, waste departing his body through one single hole. His flesh had become entirely hairless and glass-smooth. His extended middle fingers were thickened, talon-like digits with stone-hard nails, while the rest of his fingernails had molted away, as unnecessary to his current state as hair and genitals. His eyes were all pupil, save for a red ring that had eclipsed the human white. He perceived heat in gray scale, and his auditory function—an interior organ, distinct from the useless cartilage clinging to the sides of his smooth head—was greatly enhanced: he could hear the insects squirming in the dirt walls.

He relied more on animal instincts now than his failing human senses. He was intensely aware of the solar cycle, even when far beneath the planet's surface: he knew that night was arriving above. His body ran about 323 degrees Kelvin, or 50 degrees Celsius—or 120 degrees Fahrenheit. He felt, beneath the earth's surface, claustrophobia, a kinship with the darkness and the dampness, and an affinity for tight, enclosed spaces. He felt comfortable and safe underground, pulling the cold earth over himself during the day as a human would a warm blanket.

Beyond all that, he experienced a level of fellowship with the Master beyond the normal psychic link enjoyed by all the Master's children. Bolivar felt himself being groomed for some larger purpose within the growing clan. For instance, he alone knew the location of the Master's nesting place. He was aware that his consciousness was broader and deeper than the others. This he understood without forming any emotional response or independent opinion on it.

It simply was.

He was called to be at the Master's side at the time of rising.

The top cabinet doors opened out at either side. Immense hands appeared first, fingers gripping the sides of the open coffin one at a time, with the graceful coordination of spider legs. The Master pulled itself erect at the waist, clumps of old sod falling from its giant upper half back into the soil bed.

Its eyes were open. The Master was already seeing a great many things, far beyond the confines of this darkened subterranean hollow.

The solar exposure, following its encounter with the vampire hunter Setrakian, the doctor

Goodweather, and the exterminator Fet, had darkened the Master both physically and mentally. Its formerly pellucid flesh was now coarse and leathery. This skin crinkled when the Master moved, cracking and starting to peel away. It picked chips of flesh off its body like molting black feathers. The Master was missing over forty percent of its flesh now, which gave it the appearance of some horrible thing emerging from a cast of crumbling black plaster. For its flesh was not regenerating but merely the outer epidermis flaking off to reveal a lower, rawer, vascular level of skin: the dermis, and, in spots, the subcutis below, exposing the superficial fascia. In color, it ranged from gory red to a fatty yellow, like a glistening paste of beet and custard. The Master's capillary worms were more prominent all over, but especially its face, swimming just beneath the surface of its exposed dermis, rippling and racing throughout its giant body.

The Master felt the nearness of its acolyte Bolivar. It swung its massive legs over the side walls of the old cabinet, lowering itself crinklingly to the dirt floor. Some of its bed soil clung to the Master, clumps of dirt and flakes of flesh falling to the floor as it moved. Normally, a smooth-fleshed vampire slips out of soil as cleanly as a human rises from a bath of water.

The Master plucked a few larger chunks of flesh off its torso. It found that it could not move quickly and freely without shedding some of its wretched exterior. This host vehicle would not last. Bolivar, standing ready near the low burrow that was the room's exit, was an available option and an acceptable short-term physical candidate for this great honor. For Bolivar had no Dear Ones to cling to, which was one prerequisite for hosting. But Bolivar had only just begun the second stage of evolution. He was not fully mature yet.

It could wait. It would wait. The Master had much to do at present.

The Master led the way, stooping and claw-wriggling out of the chamber, swiftly clambering along the low, winding tunnels, Bolivar following right behind. It emerged into a larger chamber, nearer to the surface, the wide floor a soft bed of damp soil like that of a perfect, empty garden. Here, the ceiling was high enough even for the Master to stand erect.

As the unseen sun set above, darkness beginning its nightly rule, the soil around the Master began to stir. Limbs appeared, a small hand here, a thin leg there, like shoots of vegetation growing out of the ground. Young heads, still topped with hair, rising slowly. Some of them blank-faced, others twisted with the pain of their night rebirth.

These were the blind bus children, hatching sightless and hungry like newborn grubs. Doubly cursed by the sun—at first blinded by its occulted rays, now banished by its fatal ultraviolet spectrum—they were to become "feelers" in the Master's expanding militia: beings blessed with perception more advanced than the rest of the clan. Their special acuity would make them indispensable both as hunters and assassins.

See this.

So the Master commanded Bolivar, putting into Bolivar's mind Kelly Goodweather's point of view as she faced the old professor on the rooftop in Spanish Harlem, in the recent past.

The old man's heat signature glowed gray and cool, while the sword in his hand shone so brightly that Bolivar's nictitating eyelid lowered in a defensive squint.

Kelly escaped across the rooftops, Bolivar sharing her perspective as she leaped and ran—until she started down the side of a building.

The Master then put into Bolivar's head an animal-like perception of the building's location within the clan's ever-expanding atlas of subterranean transit.

The old man. He is yours.

IRT South Ferry Inner Loop Station

FET REACHED THE homeless encampment before nightfall. He carried the egg-timer explosive and his nail gun in a duffel bag. He ducked down below at the Bowling Green station, picking his way along the tracks toward the South Ferry encampment.

There, he struggled to locate Cray-Z's pad. Only a few items remained: a few wood shards from his pallets, and the smiling face of Mayor Koch. But it was enough to give Fet a marker. He turned and set out in the general direction of the ducts.

He heard a commotion echoing back through

the tunnel. Loud metallic banging, and a rumor of distant voices.

He pulled out his nail gun and made his way toward the loop. There he found Cray-Z, now stripped down to his dirty underwear, brown skin glistening with tunnel seepage and sweat, his ragged braid swinging behind him as he worked to pull up his ratty sofa.

Here was his dismantled home shack, the debris piled up along with the detritus of the other abandoned shacks, forming an obstruction across the tracks. The mound of refuse crested five foot high at its tallest, where he had added some broken track ties for good measure.

"Hey, brother!" called Fet. "What the hell are you doing?"

Cray-Z turned around, standing atop his junk pile like an artist in the throes of madness. He wielded a section of steel pipe in his hand. "It's time!" he yelled, as though from the summit of a mountain. "Somebody had to do something!"

Fet was a moment finding his voice. "You're gonna derail the goddamn train!"

"Now you're down with the plan!" Cray-Z responded.

Now some of the other remaining moles ambled over, witnessing Cray-Z's creation. "What have you done?" said one. His name was Caver Carl, a former trackman himself who found he could not leave the familiarity of the tunnels upon his retirement, and so returned to them like a sailor retiring to the seas. Carl wore a headlamp, the beam moving with the shaking of his head.

Cray-Z, bothered by the light beam, let out a battle cry from the top of his barricade. "I am God's fool, but they won't take me this soon!"

Caver Carl and some others moved forward, attempting to tear down the pile. "One of the trains crash, they'll drive us out of here for good!"

In an instant, Cray-Z leaped down from his pile, landing next to Fet. Fet went to him with arms outstretched, trying to calm the situation, hoping to put these folks to work for him. "Hold on everyone—"

Cray-Z wasn't in the mood for talking. He swung his steel pipe at Fet, who instinctively blocked the blow with his left forearm. The pipe cracked the bone.

Fet howled, and then, using the heavy nail gun as a club, struck Cray-Z hard across the temple. It staggered the madman, but he kept coming. Fet cracked Cray-Z in the ribs, then kicked at the calf of his right leg, dislocating his leg at the knee, finally bringing him down.

"Listen!" yelled Caver Carl.

Fet stopped and did so.

The telltale rumble. He turned and saw, down the length of the track, a dusting of light against the curve in the tunnel wall.

The 5 train was approaching its U-turn.

The other moles continued to pull at the pieces of the pile, but it was no use. Cray-Z used his pipe to get up onto his one good leg, hopping up and down.

"Fucking sinners!" he howled. "You moles

are all blind! Here they come! Now you have no choice but to fight them. Fight for your lives!"

The train bore down on them, and Fet saw that there was no time. He backed off from the impending catastrophe, the brightening train light illuminating Cray-Z's dance: a mad jig on his bent leg.

As the train blew past him, Fet caught a glimpse of the driver's face. She stared straight ahead, without expression. She had to have seen the debris. And yet she never applied the brake, she never did anything.

She had the thousand-yard-stare of a newly turned vampire.

WHAM, the train impacted the obstruction, wheels spinning, churning. The front car punched into the debris, exploding it, chewing and carrying the larger objects for some thirty feet before jumping the track. The cars lurched to the right, striking the edge of the platform at the head of the loop, still skidding, trailing a comet of sparks. The engine car of the train then wobbled the other way, the cars behind it ribboning along—the train jackknifing in the narrow track space.

The grating, metallic screech was nearly human in its outrage and its pain. Given the tunnels and their throat-like propensity for echoes, the cars stopped long before the awful sound did.

This train had many more bodies riding its exterior. Some were killed instantly—ground against and smeared along the edge of the platform. The rest rode the spectacular crash until the end. Once the cars came to a stop, they separated from the train like leeches detaching from flesh, dropping to the ground, getting their bearings.

Slowly, they turned toward the moles still standing there, staring in disbelief.

The riders walked out of the dust and smoke of the calamity, unfazed but for an odd, slinking gait. Their joints emitted a soft popping noise as they advanced.

Fet quickly went into his duffel bag, retrieving Setrakian's improvised time bomb. He felt an intense burning in the right calf and looked down. A long, thin, needle-sharp piece of debris had somehow pierced his leg, all the way through. If he pulled it loose, the bleeding would be savage—and right now, blood was the last thing he wanted to smell of. He left it painfully lodged in his muscle mass.

Closer to the tracks, Cray-Z looked on in amazement. How could so many have survived?

Then, as the riders moved closer, even Cray-Z noticed that something was missing from these people. He detected traces of humanity in their faces, but it was only that: traces. Like the glimmer of greedy humanoid intelligence one sees inside the eyes of a hungry dog.

He recognized some of them, women and men from underground. Fellow moles—except for one figure. A lanky creature, pale and bare-chested, sculpted like an ivory figurine. A few strands of hair framed an angular, handsome, yet wholly possessed face.

It was Gabriel Bolivar. His music had not permeated the under-city demographic, and yet every eye fell upon him. He stood out from the rest that much, the showman he was in life carrying over into un-death. He wore black leather pants and cowboy boots, with no shirt. Every vein, muscle, and sinew in his torso was visible beneath his delicate, translucent skin.

Flanking him were two broken females. One's arm was sliced open, a deep cut, slashing through flesh, muscle, and bone, nearly severing the limb. The cut did not bleed, but rather oozed—and not red blood, but a white substance more viscous than milk yet thinner in consistency than cream.

Caver Carl began to pray. His softly sobbing voice was so high, so full of fear, that Fet at first thought it belonged to a boy.

Bolivar pointed at the staring moles—and at once the riders were upon them.

The woman-thing ran straight at Caver Carl, knocking him back off his feet, landing on his chest, and pinning him to the ground. She smelled of moldy orange peels and spoiled meat. He tried to fend her off, but she gripped his arm and twisted it in the socket, snapping it instantly.

Her hot hand pushed at his chin with enormous strength. Carl's head was forced back to the breaking point, his neck extended and fully exposed. From his upside-down perspective, by the light of his miner's helmet, all he could see were legs and unlaced shoes and bare feet running past. A horde of creatures—reinforcements—came at them from the tunnels, a full-on invasion trampling through camp, beings clustered over twitching bodies.

A second creature joined the woman on him, tearing away his shirt in a frenzy. He felt a hard bite at his neck. Not a hinged bite—not teeth—but a puncture, followed immediately by a suction-like latching. The other clawed at the inseam of his trousers, shredding them below his groin and clamping onto the inside of his thigh.

Pain at first, a sharp burning. Then, within moments . . . numbness. The sensation was like that of a piston thumping against his muscle and flesh.

He was being drained. Carl attempted to scream, his open mouth finding no voice but only four long, hot fingers. The creature grabbed hold of his cheek from the inside, its talon-like nail slicing his gum all the way to the jawbone. Its flesh tasted salty, tangy—until it was over-whelmed by the coppery flavor of his own blood.

Fet had retreated immediately after the crash, knowing a losing battle when he saw one. The screaming was nearly unbearable, yet he had a mission to complete, and that was his focus.

He climbed backward into one of the ducts, finding there was barely enough space to accom-modate him. One advantage to fear was that the adrenaline coursing through him had the effect of dilating his pupils, and he found he could see his environs with unnatural clarity.

He unwrapped the rags and twisted the timer

one full rotation. Three minutes. One hundred eighty seconds. A soft-boiled egg.

He cursed his luck, now realizing that, with the vampire battle in the tunnel, he would have to travel deeper into the ducts used by vampires to transverse the river, but also backward, with his arm badly bruised and his leg dripping blood.

Before releasing the timer, he saw the bodies of the moles on the ground, squirming as they were consumed by clusters of vampires. They were already infected, already lost—all except for Cray-Z. He stood near a concrete pillar, watching like a blissful fool. And yet he was untouched by these dark things, unmolested as they rampaged past him.

Then Fet saw the lanky figure of Gabriel Bolivar approach Cray-Z. Cray-Z fell to his knees before the singer, the two of them outlined in smoke and dusty light, like figures in a Bible stamp.

Bolivar lay his hand upon Cray-Z's head, and the madman bowed. He then kissed the hand, praying.

Fet had seen enough. He set the device down inside a gap and took his hand off the dial . . . one . . . two . . . three . . . counting in time with the ticking as he grabbed his duffel bag and retreated backward.

Fet kept pushing back, feeling his body ease after a while, lubricated by his own flowing blood.

. . . forty . . . forty-one . . . forty-two . . .

A cluster of creatures moved toward the duct entrance, attracted by the smell of Fet's ambrosia

Fet saw their outline in the small aperture, and lost all hope.

. . . seventy-three . . . seventy-four . . . seventy-five . . .

He skidded as fast as he could, opening his duffel bag and removing his nail gun. He fired the silver nails as he retreated—screaming like a soldier emptying a machine gun into the enemy's nest.

The nails embedded deep into the cheekbone and forehead of the first charging vampire, a nicely suited man in his sixties. Fet fired again, popping the man's eye and gagging him with silver, the brad buried in the soft flesh of its throat.

The thing squealed and recoiled. Others scrambled over their fallen comrade, snaking quickly through the duct. Fet saw it approach—this one a slender woman in jogging sweats, her shoulder wounded, exposing her collarbone, scraping it against the tube walls.

. . . one hundred fifty . . . one hundred fifty-one . . . one hundred fifty-two . . .

Fet shot at the approaching creature. It kept creeping toward him even as its face was festooned with silver. Its goddamn stinger shot out of its pincushion face, fully extended, nearly touching Fet, forcing him to scramble harder, slipping on his blood, his next shot missing, the nail ricocheting past the lead vampire and burying itself in the throat of the creature behind it.

How far along was he? Fifty feet from the explosion? A hundred feet?

Not enough.

Three sticks of dynamite and a soft-fucking-boiled egg later, he would find out.

He remembered the photos of the houses with their windows all lit up inside as he kept shooting and screaming. Houses that never needed exterminators. If there was any way he could survive this, he promised himself he would light up all the windows in his apartment and go out on the street just to look back.

. . . one-seventy-six . . . one-seventy-seven . . . one-seventy—

As the explosion rose behind the creature, and the blast of heat hit Vasiliy, he felt his body pushed by the searing piston of displaced air, and a body—that of a singed vampire—hit him full-on . . . knocking him out.

As he faded into a serene void, a word out of the depths of his mind replaced the cadence of the counting in his head:

CRO . . . CRO . . .

CROATOAN

Arlington Park, Jersey City

TEN THIRTY AT NIGHT.

Alfonso Creem had been at the park an hour already, selecting a strategic spot.

He was picky that way.

The only thing he didn't like about the location was the security light above, shining down in orange. So he had his lieutenant Royal—just Royal—bust the lock on the base and pop out the plate and jam a tire iron inside. Problem solved. The light flickered out above, and Creem nodded his approval.

He took his place under the shadows. His muscular arms hung out from his sides, too big to cross over his chest. His midsection was broad and nearly square. The head of the Jersey Sapphires was a black Colombian, the son of a Brit father and a Colombian mother. The Jersey Sapphires ran every block surrounding Arlington Park. They could have the park too, if they wanted it, but it wasn't worth the trouble. The park was a criminal bazaar at night, and cleaning it out was a job for the cops and good citizens, not the Sapphires. Indeed, it was to Creem's advantage to have this dead zone here in the middle of Jersey City: a public toilet that drew the scumbags away from his blocks.

Creem had won every street corner by sheer force. He rolled in like a Sherman tank and battered the opposing force into submission. Every time he earned another corner, he celebrated by having one of his teeth capped in silver. Creem had a brilliant and intimidating smile. Silver bling dressed his fingers as well. He had chains, too, but tonight he had left his neckwear back at his crib; it's the first thing desperate people grab when they know they're about to be murdered.

Royal stood near Creem, sweating inside a fur-lined parka, an ace of spades sewn into the front of his black knit cap. "He didn't say to meet alone?"

Creem said, "Just that he wanted to parlay."

"Huh. So what's the plan?"

"His plan? No fucking idea. My plan? A nice *puto* scar." Creem used his thick thumb to mime a straight razor cutting deep across Royal's face. "I fucking hate most Mexicans, but this one 'specially."

"I wondered why the park."

Murders in the park didn't get solved. Because there was no outcry. If you were brave enough to enter A Park after dark, then you were dumb enough to die. Just in case, Creem had coated his fingertips with Crazy Glue to obscure his fingerprints, and had readied a flat razor's handle with Vaseline and bleach—just like he would with a gun handle—to avoid leaving any DNA traces.

A long, black car pulled down the street. Not quite a limousine, but something swankier than a tricked-out Cadillac. It slowed at the curb, stopped. Tinted windows stayed up. The driver didn't get out.

Royal looked at Creem. Creem looked at Royal.

The back door opened to the curb. The occupant got out, wearing sunglasses. Also a checked shirt unbuttoned over a white tank, baggy pants, new black boots. He removed his pinch-front hat, revealing a tight red do-rag beneath, and tossed the hat back onto the seat of the car.

Royal said, under his breath, "What the fuck is this?"

The *puto* crossed the sidewalk, entering through the opening in the fence. His white tank shirt glowed with what was bright in the night as he strolled over grass and dirt.

Creem didn't believe his own eyes until the dude was near enough that his collarbone tat showed plain.

SOY COMO SOY. I am what I am.

Creem said, "Am I supposed to be impressed?"

Gus Elizalde of Spanish Harlem's La Mugre gang smiled but said nothing.

The car remained idling at the curb.

Creem said, "What? You come all the way here to tell me you won the fucking lottery?"

"Sort of like that."

Creem dismissed him with a look up and down.

Gus said, "Fact, I'm here to offer you a percentage of the winning ticket."

Creem snarled, trying to figure out the Mexican's play. "What you thinking, homes? Riding that thing into my territory?"

"Everything is a dis with you, Creem," said Gus. "Why you stuck forever in Jersey City."

"You talking to the king of JC. Now who else you got with you in that sled?"

"Funny you should ask." Gus looked back with a chin nod, and the driver's door opened. Instead of a chauffeur with a cap, a large man stood out wearing a hoodie, his face obscured in shadow. He came around and stood before the front wheel, head down, waiting.

Creem said, "So you boosted a ride in from the airport. Big man."

"The old ways are over, Creem. I've seen it, man. I've seen the fucking end. Turf battles? This block-by-block shit is so two-thousand-late.

Means nothing. The only turf battle that matters now is all or nothing. Us or them."

"Them who?"

"You gotta know something's going down. And not just in the big island across the river."

"Big island? That's your problem."

"Look at this park. Where your junkies at? Crack whores? Where's the action? Dead in here. 'Cause they take the night people first."

Creem snarled. He didn't like Gus making sense. "I do know that business is down."

"Business is set to vanish, homes. There's a new drug hot on the street. Check it out. It's called human fucking blood. And it's free for the taking if you got the taste."

Royal said, "You're one of those vampire nuts. *Loco.*"

"They got my *madre* and my brother, yo. You remember Crispin?"

Gus's junkie brother. Creem said, "I remember."

"Well, you won't be seeing him around this park much anymore. But I don't grudge, Creem. Not no more. This here is a new day. I gotta set personal feelings aside. Because right now I am pulling together the best team of motherfucking hard-asses I can find."

"If you're here to talk up some shit-ass scheme to take down a bank or some shit, capitalizing on all this chaos, that's already been—"

"Looting's for amateurs. Them's day wages. I got real work, for real pay, lined up. Call in your boys, so they can hear this."

"What boys?"

"Creem. The ones set to dust me tonight, get them in here."

Creem flat-eyed Gus for a few moments. Then he whistled. Creem was a champion whistler. The silver on his teeth made for a shrill signal.

Three other Sapphires came out of the trees, hands in pockets. Gus kept his hands out and open where they could see him.

"Okay," said Creem. "Talk fast, Mex."

"I'll talk slow. You listen good."

He laid it out for them. The turf battle between the Ancients and the rogue Master.

"You been smoking," said Creem.

But Gus saw the fire in his eyes. He saw the fuse of excitement already burning. "What I am offering you is more money than you could ever clear in the powder trade. The opportunity to kill and maim at will—and never see jail for it. I am offering you a once-in-a-lifetime chance to kick unlimited ass in five boroughs. And—do the job right, we're all set for life."

"And if we don't do the job right?"

"Then I don't see how money's gonna mean shit anyway. But at least you'll have gotten your fucking rocks off, 'cause, if nothing else, this is about going out with a bang, know what I mean?"

Creem said, "Fuck, you're a little too good to be true. I need to see some green first."

Gus chuckled. "Tell you what I'm gonna do. I'm gonna show you three colors, Creem. Silver, green, and white."

He raised his hand in signal to the hooded driver. The driver went to the trunk, popped it

GUILLERMO DEL TORO AND CHUCK HOGAN

open, and retrieved two bags. He ported them through the fence opening to the meeting place, and set them down.

One was a large black duffel bag, the other a moderately sized, two-handled leather clutch.

"Who your homie?" said Creem. The driver was big, wearing heavy Doc Martens, blue jeans, and the large hoodie. Creem couldn't see the driver's face under the hood, but it was obvious this close that this guy was all wrong.

"They call him Mr. Quinlan," said Gus.

A scream arose from the other end of the park—a man's scream, more terrible to the ears than a woman's scream. The others turned.

Gus said, "Let's hurry. First—the silver."

He knelt and drew the zipper across the duffel. There wasn't much light. Gus pulled out the long gun and felt the Sapphires reach for theirs. Gus flipped the switch on the barrel-mounted lamp, thinking it was a normal incandescent bulb, but it was ultraviolet. Of course.

He used the inky-purple light to show the rest of the weapons. A crossbow, its bolt load tipped with a silver impact charge. A flat, fan-shaped silver blade with a curved wooden handle. A sword fashioned like a wide-bladed scimitar with a generous curve and a rugged, leather-bound handle.

Gus said, "You like silver, Creem, don't you?"

The exotic-looking weaponry piqued Creem's interest. But he was still wary of the driver, Quinlan. "All right. What about the green?"

Quinlan opened the handles of the leather bag.

Filled with bundles of cash, anti-counterfeiting threads glowing under the indigo eye of Gus's UV light.

Creem started to reach into the bag—then stopped. He noticed Quinlan's hands gripping the bag handles. Most of his fingernails were gone, his flesh entirely smooth. But the fucked-up thing was his middle fingers. Twice as long as the rest of the digits, and crooked at the end—so much so that the tip curled around his palm to the side of his hand.

Another scream split the night, followed by a kind of growl. Quinlan closed the bag, looking forward into the trees. He handed the money bag to Gus, trading him for the long gun. Then, with unbelievable power and speed, he went sprinting into the trees.

Creem said, "What the . . . ?"

If there was a path, this Quinlan ignored it. The gangsters heard branches cracking.

Gus slung the weapons bag onto his shoulder. "Come on. You don't want to miss this."

He was easy to follow, because Quinlan had cleared a path of downed branches, pointing the way straight ahead, weaving only for tree trunks. They hustled along, coming upon Quinlan in a clearing on the other side, finding him standing quietly with the gun cradled against his chest.

His hood had fallen back. Creem, huffing, saw the driver's smooth bald head from behind. In the darkness, it looked like the guy had no ears. Creem came around to see his face better—and the human tank shivered like a little flower in a storm.

The thing called Quinlan had no ears and barely any nose left. A thick throat. Translucent skin, nearly iridescent. And blood-red eyes—the brightest eyes Creem had ever seen—set deep within his pale, smooth head.

Just then a figure broke from the upper branches, dropping to the ground with ease and loping across the clearing. Quinlan sprinted out to intercept it like a cougar tracking a gazelle. They collided, Quinlan dropping his shoulder for an open-field hit.

The figure went down sprawling with a squeal, rolling hard—before popping right back up.

In an instant, Quinlan turned the barrel light on the figure. The figure hissed and flailed back, the torture in its face evident even from that distance. Then Quinlan pulled the trigger. An exploding cone of bright silver buckshot obliterated the figure's head.

Only—the figure didn't die like a man dies. A white substance geysered out from its neck trunk and it tucked in its arms and collapsed to the ground.

Quinlan turned his head fast—even before the next figure darted from the trees. A female this time, racing away from Quinlan, toward the others. *At* the others. Gus pulled the scimitar from the bag. The female—dressed in tatters like the filthiest crack whore you've ever seen, except that she was nimble and her eyes shone red—reeled back from the sight of the weapon, but too late. With a single, clean move, Gus connected with the tops of her shoulders and her neck, her head falling one way, her body the other. When it all settled to the ground, a pasty-white liquid oozed out of her wounds.

"And there's the white," Gus said.

Quinlan returned to them, pumping the long gun and raising his thick cotton hood back over his head.

"Okay, yeah," said Creem, dancing from side to side like a kid who had to go to the bathroom on Christmas morning. "Yeah, I'd say we're fucking in."

The Flatlands

USING A STRAIGHT razor taken from the pawnshop, Eph shaved half his face before losing interest. He zoned out, staring into the mirror over the sink of milky water, his right cheek still covered in foam.

He was thinking of the book—the *Occido Lumen*—and how everything was going against him. Palmer and his fortune. Blocking every move they could make. What would become of them—of Zack—if he failed?

The edge of the razor drew blood. A thin nick turning red and flowing. He looked at the blade with the smear of blood on the steel, and drifted back eleven years to Zack's birth.

Following one miscarriage and a stillbirth at twenty-nine weeks, Kelly had been on two months' bed rest with Zack before going into labor. She had a specific birth plan going in: no epidural or drugs of any kind, no cesarean section. Ten hours later, there was little progression. Her doctor suggested Pitocin in order to speed things up, but Kelly declined, sticking to her plan. Eight hours of labor later, she relented, and the Pitocin drip was begun. Two hours after that, after enduring almost a full day of painful contractions, she finally consented to an epidural. The Pitocin dose was gradually increased until it was as high as the baby's heart rate would allow.

At the twenty-seventh hour, her doctor offered her the option of a cesarean, but Kelly refused. Having given in on every other point, she held out for natural birth. The fetus's heart monitor showed that it was doing okay, her cervix had dilated to eight centimeters, and Kelly was intent on pushing her baby out into the world.

But five hours later, despite a vigorous belly-massage from a veteran nurse, the baby remained stubbornly sideways, and Kelly's cervix was stuck at eight. The pain of the contractions was registering now, despite the successful epidural. Kelly's doctor rolled a stool over to her bedside, again offered her a cesarean. This time Kelly accepted.

Eph gowned up and accompanied her to the glowing white operating room through the double doors at the end of the hall. The fetal heart monitor reassured him with its swift, metronomic *tock-tock-tock*. The attending nurse swabbed Kelly's swollen belly with yellow-brown antiseptic, and then the obstetrician sliced left to right low on her abdomen with confident, broad strokes: the fascia was parted, then the twin vertical belts of the beefy abdominal muscle, and then the thin peritoneum membrane, revealing the thick, plum wall of the uterus. The surgeon switched to bandage scissors so as to minimize any risk of lacerating the fetus, and made the final incision.

Gloved hands reached in and pulled out a brand-new human being—but Zack was not yet born. He was "in the caul," as they say; that is, still surrounded by the filmy, intact amniotic sac. It ballooned like a bubble, an opaque membrane encircling the fetal infant like a nylon egg. Zack was still, in that moment, feeding off Kelly, still receiving nutrients and oxygen through the umbilical cord. The obstetrician and attending nurses worked to retain their professional poise, but Kelly and Eph both felt their apparent alarm. Only later would Eph learn that caul babies occur in fewer than one in a thousand births, with the number rising into the tens of thousands for babies not born prematurely.

This strange moment lingered, the unborn baby still tethered to his exhausted mother, delivered and yet unborn. Then the membrane spontaneously ruptured, peeling back from Zack's head to reveal his glistening face. Another moment of suspended time . . . and then he cried out, and was placed dripping onto Kelly's chest.

Tension lingered in the operating room, mixed with obvious joy, Kelly pulling at Zack's feet and hands to count the digits. She searched him thoroughly for signs of deformity, and found only joy. He was eight pounds even, bald as a lump of bread dough and just as pale. His Apgar score was eight after two minutes, nine after five minutes.

Healthy baby.

Kelly, however, experienced a big letdown postpartum. Nothing as deep and debilitating as true depression, but a dark funk nonetheless. The marathon labor was so debilitating that her milk did not come in, which, combined with her abandoned birth plan, left her feeling like a failure. At one point, Kelly told Eph that she felt she had let *him* down, which mystified him. She felt corrupted inside. Everything in life had come so easily, to both of them, before this.

Once she got better—once she embraced the golden boy who was her newborn son—she never let Zack go. She became, for a time, obsessed with the caul birth, researching its significance. Some sources claimed the oddity was an omen of good luck, even forecasting greatness. Other legends indicated that caul-bearers, as they were known, were clairvoyant, would never drown, and had been marked by angels with shielded souls. She looked for meaning in literature, citing various fictional caul-bearers, such as David Copperfield and the little boy in *The Shining*. Famous men in real life, such as Sigmund Freud, Lord Byron, and Napoleon Bonaparte. In time, she came to discount all negative associations—in fact, in certain European countries it was said that a child born with a caul might be cursed—countering her own unfortunate feelings of inadequacy with the determination that her boy, this creation of hers, was exceptional.

It was these impulses that, over time, poisoned her relationship with Eph, leading to a divorce he never wanted, and the ensuing custody battle: a battle that had, since her turning, morphed into a life-or-death struggle. Kelly had decided that if she couldn't be perfect for so exacting a man, then she would be nothing to him. And so it was that Eph's personal downfall—his drinking— secretly thrilled her at the same time as it terri-fied her. Kelly's awful wish had come true. For it showed that even Ephraim Goodweather could not live up to his own exacting standards.

Eph smiled derisively at his half-shaven self in the mirror. He reached for his bottle of apri-cot schnapps and toasted his fucking perfection, downing two sweetly harsh gulps.

"You don't need to do that."

Nora had entered, easing the bathroom door shut behind her. She was barefoot, having changed into fresh jeans and a loose T-shirt, her dark hair clipped up in back of her head.

Eph addressed her mirror reflection. "We're outmoded, you know. Our time has passed. The twentieth century was viruses. The twenty-first? Vampires." He drank again, as proof that he was all right with it, and demonstrating that no ra-tional argument could dissuade him. "I don't get how you don't drink. This is exactly what booze was made for. The only way to swallow this new reality is by chasing it with some of the good stuff." Another drink, then he looked again at the label. "If only I had some good stuff."

"I don't like you like this."

"I am what experts refer to as a 'high-functioning alcoholic.' Or I could go around hiding it, if you prefer."

She crossed her arms, leaning sideways against the wall, staring at his back and knowing she was getting nowhere. "It's only a matter of time, you know. Before Kelly's blood-yearning leads her back here, to Zack. And that means, through her, the Master. Leading him straight to Setrakian."

If the bottle had been empty, Eph might have whipped it against the wall. "It's fucking insanity. But it's *real*. I've never had a nightmare that's even come *close* to this."

"I'm saying I think you need to get Zack away from here."

Eph nodded, both hands gripping the edge of the sink. "I know. I've been slowly coming around to that determination myself."

"And I think you need to go with him."

Eph considered it a moment, he truly did, before turning from the mirror to face her. "Is this like when the first lieutenant informs the captain he's not fit for duty?"

Nora said, "This is like when someone cares enough for you that they are afraid you will hurt yourself. It's best for him—and better for you."

That disarmed him. "I can't leave you here in my place, Nora. We both know the city is falling. New York City is over. Better it falls on me than on you."

"That's bullshit barroom talk."

"You are right about one thing. With Zack here, I can't fully commit myself to this fight. He needs to go. I need to know he's out of here, he's safe. There is this place, in Vermont—"

"I am not leaving."

Eph took a breath. "Just listen."

"I am not leaving, Eph. You think you're doing the chivalrous thing, when, in fact, you are insulting me. This is my city more than it is yours. Zack is a great kid, you know I think that, but I am not here to do the women's work and watch the children and lay out your clothes. I am a medical scientist just like you."

"I know all that, believe me. I was thinking about your mother."

That stopped her in her tracks. Nora's lips remained parted, ready to fire back, but his words had stolen the breath from her mouth.

"I know she's not well," he went on. "She's in early-phase dementia, and I know she weighs on your mind constantly, same as Zack does on mine. This is your chance to get her out too. I'm trying to tell you that Kelly's folks had this place on a mountain in Vermont—"

"I can do more good here."

"Can you, though? I mean—can I? I don't even know. What's most important now? Survival, I'd say. That's the absolute best we can hope for. At least this way, one of us will be safe. And I know it's not what you want. And I know it's a ton to ask of you. You're right—were this a normal viral pandemic, you and I would be the most essential people in this city. We would be at the crux of this thing—for all the right reasons. As it is now, this strain has leapfrogged our expertise entirely. The world doesn't need us anymore, Nora. It doesn't need doctors or scientists. It needs exorcists. It needs Abraham Setrakian." Eph crossed to her. "I know just enough to be dangerous. And so—dangerous I must be."

That brought her forward from the wall. "What exactly is that supposed to mean?"

"I'm expendable. Or, at least, as expendable as the next man. Unless the next man in question is an aging pawnbroker with a bad heart. Hell— Fet brings much more to this fight than I do now. He's more valuable to the old man than I am."

"I don't like the way you're talking."

He was impatient that she accept the realities as he understood them. That he make her understand. "I want to fight. I want to give it my all. But I can't, not with Kelly coming after the people I care about most. I need to know that my Dear Ones are safe. That means Zack. And that means you."

He reached for her hand. Their fingers intertwined. The sensation was profound, and it occurred to Eph: how many days now had it been since he had experienced a simple physical contact with another person?

"What is it you plan to do?" asked Nora.

He knit his fingers more firmly into hers, exploring the fit as he reaffirmed the plan taking form in his mind. Dangerous and desperate, but effective. Maybe a game-changer.

He answered, "Simply to be useful."

He turned away, trying to reach back for the bottle on the sink edge, but she gripped his arm and pulled him back toward her. "Leave it there," she said. "Please." Her tea-brown eyes were so beautiful, so sad—so human. "You don't need it."

"But I want it. And it wants me."

He wanted to turn but she held him fast. "Kelly couldn't get you to stop?"

Eph thought about that. "You know, I'm not sure she ever really tried."

Nora reached for his face, her hand touching first his bristly, unshaven cheek, then the smooth side, stroking it gently with the backs of her fingers. The contact melted them both.

"I could make you stop," she said, very close to his face.

She kissed the rough side first. Then he met her lips and experienced a surge of hope and passion so powerful, it was like a first-time embrace. Everything about their previous two sexual encounters came swarming back to him in a hot, anticipatory rush, and yet it was the fundamental human contact that supercharged the exchange. That which had been missing was now craved.

Exhausted, strung out, and utterly unprepared, they clung to each other as Eph pressed Nora back against the tile wall, his hands wanting only her flesh. In the face of such terror and dehumanization, human passion itself was an act of defiance.

OCCIDO LUMEN:

THE STORY OF THE BOOK

THE BROWN-SKINNED BROKER IN THE BLACK velvet Nehru jacket twisted a blue opal ring around the base of his pinkie finger as he strolled the canal. "I have never met Mynheer Blaak, mind you. He prefers it that way."

Setrakian walked alongside the broker. Setrakian was traveling with a Belgian passport, under the name Roald Pirk, his occupation listed as "antique bookseller." The document was an expert forgery.

The year was 1972. Setrakian was forty-six years old.

"Though I can assure you he is very wealthy," the broker continued. "Do you like money very much, Monsieur Pirk?"

"I do."

"Then you will like Mynheer Blaak very much. This volume he seeks, he will pay you quite handsomely. I am authorized to say that he will match your price, which, itself, I would characterize as aggressive. This makes you happy?"

"Yes."

"As it should. You are fortunate indeed to have acquired such a rare volume. I am sure you are aware of its provenance. You are not a superstitious man?"

"In fact, I am. By trade."

"Ah. And that is why you have chosen to part with it? Myself, I think of this volume as the book version of 'The Bottle Imp.' You are familiar with the tale?"

"Stevenson, wasn't it?"

"Indeed. Oh, I hope you aren't thinking that I am testing your knowledge of literature in order to gauge your bona fides. I reference Stevenson only because I recently brokered the sale of an extremely rare edition of *The Master of Ballantrae*. But in 'Imp,' as you evidently remember, the accursed bottle must be sold each time for less than it was purchased. Not so with this volume. No, no. Quite the opposite."

The broker's eyes flashed with interest at one of the brightly lit display windows they strolled past. Unlike most of the other showcases along De Wallen, the red-light district of Amsterdam, the occupant of this particular window was a ladyboy, not the usual female prostitute.

The broker smoothed his mustache and redirected his eyes to the brick-paved street. "In any event," he continued, "the book has a troubling legacy. I myself will not handle it. Mynheer Blaak is an avid collector, a connoisseur of the first rank. His tastes run to the discriminating and the obscure, and his checks always clear. But I feel it is only fair to warn you, there have been a few attempts at fraud."

"I see."

"I, of course, can accept no responsibility for what became of these crooked sellers. Though I must say, Mynheer Blaak's interest in the volume is keen, because he has paid half of my commission on every unsuccessful transaction. In order that I might continue my search and keep potential suitors arriving at his door, so to speak."

The broker casually pulled out a pair of fine white cotton gloves and fitted them over his manicured hands.

"If you will forgive me," said Setrakian, "I did not journey to Amsterdam to walk its beautiful canals. I am a superstitious man, as I stated, and I should like to unload myself of the burden of such a valuable book at the earliest convenience. To be frank, I am even more concerned about robbers than curses."

"I see, yes. You are a practical man."

"Where and when will Mynheer Blaak be available to conduct this transaction?"

"The book is with you, then?"

Setrakian nodded. "It is here."

The broker pointed to the twin-handled, twin-buckled portmanteau of stiff, black leather in Setrakian's hand. "On your person?"

"No, much too risky." Setrakian moved the suitcase from one hand to the other, hoping to signal otherwise. "But it is here. In Amsterdam. It is near."

"Please forgive my boldness then. But, if you are indeed in possession of the *Lumen* then you are familiar with its content. Its raison d'être, yes?"

Setrakian stopped. For the first time he noticed they had wandered off the crowded streets and were now in a narrow alley with no one in sight. The broker folded his arms behind his back as if in casual conversation.

"I do," said Setrakian. "But it would be foolish for me to divulge much."

"Indeed," said the broker. "And we don't expect you to do so but—could you effectively summarize your impressions of it? A few words if you would."

Setrakian perceived a metallic flash behind the broker's back—or was it one of the man's gloved hands? Either way, Setrakian felt no fear. He had prepared for this.

"Mal'akh Elohim. *Messengers of God.* Angels. Archangels. In this case, Fallen Ones. And their corrupt lineage on this Earth."

The broker's eyes flared a moment, then were still. "Wonderful. Well, Mynheer Blaak is most interested to meet you, and will be in contact very soon."

The broker offered Setrakian a white-gloved

hand. Setrakian wore black gloves, and the broker certainly felt the crooked digits of his hand as they shook—but, aside from an impolite stiffening, did not otherwise react. Setrakian said, "Shall I give you my local address?"

The broker waved his gloved hand brusquely. "I am to know nothing. Monsieur, I wish you every success." He was starting away, back the way they came.

"But how will he contact me?" asked Setrakian, after him.

"I know only that he will," the broker responded over a velvet-lined shoulder. "A very good evening to you, Monsieur Pirk."

Setrakian watched the dapper man walk on, long enough to see him turn in toward the window they had passed and knock pleasantly. Setrakian turned up the collar of his overcoat and walked west, away from the inky water of the canals toward the Dam Platz.

Amsterdam, being a city of canals, was an unusual residence for a *strigoi*, forbidden by nature to cross over moving water. But all his years spent in pursuit of the Nazi doctor Werner Dreverhaven, the camp physician at Treblinka, had led Setrakian into a network of underground antique booksellers. That, in turn, had put him on the path to the object of Dreverhaven's obsession, this extraordinarily rare Latin translation of an obscure Mesopotamian text.

De Wallen was known more for its macabre mix of drugs, coffee bars, sex clubs, brothels, and window girls and boys. But the narrow alleys and canals of this port city were also home to a small but highly influential group of antique book merchants who traded manuscripts all over the world.

Setrakian had learned that Dreverhaven—under the guise of a bibliophile named Jan-Piet Blaak—had fled to the Low Countries in the years following the war, traveling throughout Belgium until the early 1950s, crossing into the Netherlands and settling in Amsterdam in 1955. In De Wallen, he could move freely at night, along paths proscribed by the waterways, and burrow undetected during the day. The canals discouraged his staying there, but apparently the lure of the bibliophile trade—and the *Occido Lumen* in particular—was too seductive. He had established a nest here, and made the city his permanent home.

The middle of the town was island-like, radiating from the Dam Platz, surrounded in part, but not bisected by, the canals. Setrakian walked past three-hundred-year-old gabled buildings, the fragrance of hash smoke wafting out the windows with American folk music. A young woman rushed past, hobbling in one broken heel, late for a night of work, her gartered legs and fishnet stockings showing beneath the hem of a coat of faux mink.

Setrakian came upon two pigeons on the cobblestones, who did not alight at his approach. He slowed and looked to see what had captured their interest.

The pigeons were picking apart a gutter rat.

"I am told you have the *Lumen*?"

Setrakian stiffened. The presence was very near—in fact, right behind him. But the voice originated inside his head.

Setrakian half-turned, frightened. "Mynheer Blaak?"

He was mistaken. There was no one behind him.

"Monsieur Pirk, I presume?"

Setrakian jerked to his right. In the shadowy entrance to an alleyway stood a portly figure dressed in a long, formal coat and a top hat, supporting himself with a thin, metal-tipped cane.

Setrakian swallowed his adrenaline, his anticipation, his fear. "How did you ever find me, sir?"

"The book. That is all that matters. Is it in your possession, Pirk?"

"I . . . I have it near."

"Where is your hotel?"

"I have rented a flat near the station. If you like, I would be happy to conduct our transaction there—"

"I am afraid I cannot travel that far conveniently, for I have a bad case of the gout."

Setrakian turned more fully toward the shadowed being. There were a few people out in the square, and he dared to take a step toward Dreverhaven, in the manner of an unsuspecting man. He did not smell the usual earthy musk of the *strigoi*, though the hash smoke acted on the night like a perfume. "What would you suggest, then? I would very much like to conclude this sale this evening."

"And yet, you would have to return to your flat first."

"Yes. I guess I would."

"Hmm." The figure ventured forward a step, tapping the metal toe of its cane on a cobblestone. Wings fluttered, the pigeons taking flight behind Setrakian. Blaak said, "I wonder why a man traveling in an unfamiliar city would entrust such a valuable article to his flat rather than the security of his own person."

Setrakian switched his portmanteau from one hand to the other. "Your point?"

"I do not believe a true collector would risk allowing such a precious item out of his sight. Or his grip."

Setrakian said, "There are thieves about."

"And thieves within. If indeed you want to relieve yourself of the burden of this cursed artifact for a premium price, you will now follow me, Pirk. My residence is just a few paces this way."

Dreverhaven turned and started into the alley, using the cane but not reliant upon it. Setrakian steadied himself, licking his lips and feeling the bristles of his disguising beard as he followed the undead war criminal into the stone alleyway.

The only time Setrakian was allowed outside Treblinka's camouflaged barbwire fences was to work on Dreverhaven's library. Herr Doktor maintained a house just a few minutes' drive from the camp, workers transported there one at a time by a three-man squad of armed Ukrainian guards. Setrakian had little contact with Drever-haven at the house, and, much more fortunately, no contact with him whatsoever inside the camp surgery, where Dreverhaven sought to satisfy his medical and scientific curiosity in the manner of an indulged boy left alone to cut worms in half and burn the wings off flies.

Dreverhaven was a bibliophile even then, using the spoils of war and genocide—gold and dia-monds stolen from the walking dead—to spend outrageous sums on rare texts from Poland, France, Great Britain, and Italy, appropriated with dubious provenance during the black market chaos of the war years. Setrakian had been or-dered to do finish work on a two-room library of rich oak, complete with a rolling iron ladder and a stained-glass window portraying the rod of Asclepius. Often confused with the caduceus, the Asclepius image of a serpent or long worm coiled about a staff is the symbol for medicine and doc-tors. But the head of the staff on Dreverhaven's stained-glass representation depicted a death's head, the symbol of the Nazi SS.

Dreverhaven personally inspected Setrakian's craftsmanship once, his blue eyes crystal-cold as his fingers traced the underside of the shelves, seeking out any rough spots. He praised the young Jew with a nod and dismissed him.

They met one more time, when Setrakian faced the "Burning Hole," the doctor overseeing the slaughter with the same cold blue eyes. They did not recognize Setrakian then: too many faces, all indistinguishable to him. Still, the experimenter was busy, an assistant timing the interlude between the gunshot entering the back of the head and the last agonal twitching of the victim.

Setrakian's scholarship in the folklore and the occult history of vampires dovetailed with his hunt for the camp Nazis in his search for the ancient text known as *Occido Lumen*.

Setrakian gave "Blaak" plenty of leeway, trailing him by three paces, just out of stinger range. Dreverhaven walked on with his cane, apparently unconcerned about the vulnerability of having a stranger at his back. Perhaps he laid his trust in the many pedestrians circling the Wallen at night, their presence discouraging any attack. Or perhaps he merely *wanted* to give the impression of guilelessness.

In other words, perhaps the cat was acting like a mouse.

Between two red-lit window girls, Dreverhaven turned a key in a door lock, and Setrakian followed him up a red-carpeted flight of stairs. Dreverhaven had the top two floors, handsomely decorated if not well-lived-in. The bulb wattage was kept low, downturned lamps shining dimly onto soft rugs. The front windows faced east. They lacked heavy shades. There were no back windows, and, in sizing up the room dimensions, Setrakian determined them to be too narrow. He remembered, at once, harboring this same suspicion at his house near Treblinka—a suspicion informed by camp rumors of a secret examining room at Dreverhaven's house, a hidden surgery.

Dreverhaven moved to a lit table, upon which he rested his cane. On a porcelain tray, Setrakian recognized the paperwork he had earlier provided the broker: provenance documents establishing a plausible link to the 1911 Marseilles auction, all expensive forgeries.

Dreverhaven removed his hat and placed it on a table, yet still he did not turn around. "May I interest you in an aperitif?"

"Regrettably, no," answered Setrakian, undoing the twin buckles on his portmanteau while leaving the top clasp closed. "Travel upsets my digestive system."

"Ah. Mine is ironclad."

"Please don't deny yourself on my account."

Dreverhaven turned around, slowly, in the gloom. "I couldn't, Monsieur Pirk. It is my practice never to drink alone."

Instead of the time-worn *strigoi* Setrakian expected, he was stunned—though he tried to hide it—to find Dreverhaven looking exactly as he had decades before. Those same crystalline eyes. Raven-black hair falling over the back of his neck. Setrakian tasted a pang of acid, but he had little reason to fear: Dreverhaven had not recognized him at the pit, and surely would not recognize him now, more than a quarter century later.

"So," Dreverhaven said. "Let us consummate our happy transaction then."

Setrakian's greatest test of will involved masking his amazement at the vampire's speech. Or, more accurately, his play at speech. The vampire communicated in the usual telepathic manner, "speaking" directly into Setrakian's head—but it had learned to manipulate its useless lips in a pantomime of human speech. Setrakian now understood how, in this manner, "Jan-Piet Blaak" moved about nocturnal Amsterdam without fear of discovery.

Setrakian scanned the room for another way out. He needed to know the *strigoi* was trapped before springing on him. He had come too far to allow Dreverhaven to slip free of his grasp.

Setrakian said, "Am I to understand, then, that you have no concerns about the book, given the misfortune that seems to befall those who possess it?"

Dreverhaven stood with his hands behind his back. "I am a man who embraces the accursed, Monsieur Pirk. And besides—it seems no misfortune has befallen you yet."

"No . . . not yet," lied Setrakian. "And why this book, if I may ask?"

"A scholarly interest, if you will. You might think of me as a broker myself. In fact, I have undertaken this global search for another interested party. The book is rare indeed, not having surfaced in more than half a century. Many believe that the sole remaining edition was destroyed. But—according to your papers—perhaps it has survived. Or there is a second edition. You are prepared to produce it now?"

"I am. First, I should like to see payment."

"Ah. Naturally. In the case on the corner chair behind you."

Setrakian moved laterally, with a casualness he did not feel, finding the latch with his finger and opening the top. The case was filled with banded guilders.

"Very good," said Setrakian.

"Trading paper for paper, Monsieur Pirk. Now if you will reciprocate?"

Setrakian left the case open and returned to his portmanteau. He undid the clasp, one eye on Dreverhaven the entire time. "You might know, it has a very unusual binding."

"I am aware of that, yes."

"Though I am assured it is only partially responsible for the book's outrageous price."

"May I remind you, Monsieur, that you set the price. And do not judge a book by its cover. As with most clichés, that is good advice often ignored."

Setrakian carried the portmanteau to the table containing the papers of provenance. He pulled open the top under the faint lamp light, then withdrew. "As you will, sir."

"Please," said the vampire. "I should like you to remove it. I insist."

"Very well."

Setrakian returned to the bag and reached inside with his black-gloved hands. He pulled out the book, which was bound in silver and fronted and backed with smooth silver plates.

He offered it to Dreverhaven. The vampire's eyes narrowed, glowing.

Setrakian took a step toward him. "You would like to inspect it, of course?"

"Set it down on that table, Monsieur."

"That table? But the light is so much more favorable over here."

"You will please set it down on that table."

Setrakian did not immediately comply. He remained still, the heavy silver book in his hands. "But you must want to examine it."

Dreverhaven's eyes rose from the silver cover of the tome to take in Setrakian's face. "Your beard, Monsieur Pirk. It obscures your face. It gives you a Hebraic mien."

"Is that right? I take it you don't like Jews."

"They don't like me. Your scent, Pirk—it is familiar."

"Why don't you take a closer look at this book."

"I do not need to. It is a fake."

"Perhaps. Perhaps, indeed. But the silver—I can assure you that the silver is quite real."

Setrakian advanced on Dreverhaven, the book held out in front of him. Dreverhaven backed off, then slowed. "Your hands," he said. "You are crippled." Dreverhaven's eyes went back to Setrakian's face. "The woodworker. So it *is* you."

Setrakian swept open his coat, removing from the interior left fold a sword with a silver blade of modest size. "You have become indolent, Herr Doktor."

Dreverhaven lashed out with his stinger. Not full-length, merely a feint, the bloated vampire leaping backward against the wall, and then quickly down again.

Setrakian anticipated the ploy. Indeed, the

doctor was considerably less agile than many others Setrakian had encountered. Setrakian stood fast with his back to the windows, the vampire's only escape.

"You are too slow, doctor," Setrakian said. "Your hunting here has been too easy."

Dreverhaven hissed. Concern showed in the beast's eyes as the heat of exertion began to melt its facial cosmetics.

Dreverhaven glanced at the door, but Setrakian wasn't buying. These creatures always built in an emergency exit. Even a bloated tick like Dreverhaven.

Setrakian feigned an attack, keeping the *strigoi* off-balance, forcing him to react. Dreverhaven snapped out his stinger, another aborted thrust. Setrakian responded with a quick sweep of his blade, which would have lopped it off at full length.

Dreverhaven made his break then, rushing laterally along the back bookcases, but Setrakian was just as fast. He still held the book in one hand, and hurled it at the fat vampire, the creature recoiling from its toxic silver. Then Setrakian was upon him.

He held the point of his silver blade at Dreverhaven's upper throat. The vampire's head tipped back, its crown resting against the spines of his precious books along the upper shelf, his eyes staring at Setrakian.

The silver weakened him, keeping his stinger in check. Setrakian went into his deepest coat pocket—it was lead-lined—and removed a band of thick silver baubles wrapped in a mesh of fine steel, strung along a length of cable.

The vampire's eyes widened, but it was unable to move as Setrakian lay the necklace over its head, resting it upon the creature's shoulders.

The silver collar weighed on the *strigoi* like a chain of hundred-pound stones. Setrakian pulled over a chair just in time for Dreverhaven to collapse into it, keeping the vampire from falling to the floor. The creature's head dipped to one side, its hands shivering helplessly in its lap.

Setrakian picked up the book—it was, in fact, a sixth-edition copy of Darwin's *Origin of the Species*, backed and bound in Britannia silver—and dropped it back into his portmanteau. Sword in hand, he returned to the bookcase toward which the desperate Dreverhaven had lunged.

After some careful searching, wary of booby-traps, Setrakian found the trigger volume. He heard a click and felt the shelf unit give, and then shoved open the swinging wall on its rotating axis.

The smell met him first. Dreverhaven's rear quarters were windowless and unventilated, a nest of discarded books and trash and reeking rags. But this was not the source of the most offensive stench. That came from the top floor, accessible via a blood-spattered staircase.

An operating theater, a stainless-steel table set in black tile seemingly grouted in caked human blood. Decades of grime and gore covered every surface, flies buzzing angrily around a blood-smeared meat refrigerator in the corner.

Setrakian held his breath and opened the fridge, because he had to. It contained only items of perversion, nothing of real interest. No information to further Setrakian's quest. Setrakian realized he was becoming inured to depravity and butchering.

He returned to the creature suffering in the chair. Dreverhaven's face had by now melted away, unveiling the *strigoi* beneath. Setrakian stepped to the windows, dawn just beginning to filter in, soon to trumpet into the apartment, cleaning it of darkness and of vampires.

"How I dreaded each dawn in the camp," said Setrakian. "The start of another day in the death farm. I did not fear death, but I did not choose it either. I chose survival. And in doing so, I chose dread."

I am happy to die.

Setrakian looked at Dreverhaven. The *strigoi* no longer bothered with the ruse of moving his lips.

All my lusts have long since been satisfied. I have gone as far as one can go in this life, man or beast. I hunger for nothing any longer. Repetition only extinguishes pleasure.

"The book," said Setrakian, daringly close to Dreverhaven. "It no longer exists."

It does exist. But only a fool would dare to pursue it. Pursuing the Occido Lumen *means you are pursuing the Master. You might be able to take a tired acolyte like myself, but if you go against him, the odds will certainly be against you. As they were against your dear wife.*

So indeed the vampire had a little bit of perversion left in him. He still possessed the capacity, however small and vain, for sick pleasure. The vampire's gaze never left Setrakian's.

Morning was upon them now, the sun appearing at an angle through the windows. Setrakian stood and suddenly grasped the back of Dreverhaven's chair, tipping it onto its hind legs and dragging it through the bookcase to the hidden rear quarters, leaving twin scores in the wood floor.

"Sunlight," Setrakian declared, "is too good for you, Herr Doktor."

The *strigoi* stared at him, eyes full of anticipation. Here, finally for him, was the unexpected. Dreverhaven longed to be part of any perversion, no matter the role he might play.

Setrakian remained in tight control of his rage.

"Immortality is no friend to the perverse, you say?" Setrakian put his shoulder to the bookshelf, sealing out the sun. "Then immortality you shall enjoy."

That's it, woodworker. There is your passion, Jew. What have you in mind?

The plan took three days. For seventy-two hours, Setrakian worked nonstop in a vengeful daze. Dismembering the *strigoi* upon Dreverhaven's own operating table, severing and cauterizing all four stumps, was the most dangerous part. He then procured lead tulip planters in order to fashion a dirt-less coffin for the silver-necklaced *strigoi*, in order to cut off the vampire from communication with the Master. Into the sarcophagus he packed the abomination and its severed limbs. Setrakian chartered a small boat and loaded the planter onto it. Then he sailed alone deep into the North Sea. After a struggle, he managed to put the box overboard without sinking the boat in the process—thereby stranding the creature between land masses, safe from the killing sun and yet impotent for all eternity.

Not until the box sank to the ocean floor did Dreverhaven's taunting voice finally leave Setrakian's mind, like a madness finding its cure. Setrakian looked at his crooked fingers, bruised and bleeding, stinging with the salt water—and clenched them into tangled fists.

He was indeed going the way of madness. It was time to go underground, he realized, just as the *strigoi* had. To continue his work in private, and to await his chance.

His chance at the book. At the Master.

It was time to repair to America.

The Master—Part II

THE MASTER WAS, above all things, compulsive in both action and thought. The Master had considered every potential permutation of the plan. It felt vaguely anxious for this all to come to fruition, but one thing the Master did not lack was conviction.

The Ancients would be exterminated all at once, and in a matter of hours.

They would not even see it coming. How could they? After all, hadn't the Master orchestrated the demise of one of them, along with six serfs, some years ago in the city of Sofia, Bulgaria? The Master itself had shared in the pain of the anguish of death at the very moment it occurred, feeling the maelstrom pull of the darkness—the implacable nothing—and savoring it.

On the 26th of April, 1986, several hundred meters below at the center of the Bulgarian city, a solar flash—a fission approximating the power of the sun—occurred inside a vaulted cellar within fifteen-foot-thick concrete walls. The city above was shaken by a deep rumble and a seismic movement, its epicenter tracked to Pirotska Street—but there were no injuries, and very little damage to property.

The event had been a mere bleep in the news, barely worth mentioning. It was to become completely overshadowed by the meltdown of the reactor at Chernobyl, and yet, in a manner unknown to most, intimately related to it.

Of the original seven, the Master had remained the most ambitious, the hungriest—and, in a sense, the youngest. This was only natural. The Master was the last one to arise, and from whence it was created was the mouth, the throat, *the thirst*.

Divided by this thirst, the others were scattered and hidden. Concealed, yet connected.

These notions buzzed inside the great consciousness of the Master. Its thoughts wandered to the time the Master first visited Armageddon on this Earth—to cities long forgotten, with pillars of alabaster and floors of polished onyx.

To the first time it had tasted blood.

Quickly, the Master reasserted control over its thoughts. Memories were a dangerous thing. They individuated the Master's mind, and when that happened, even in this protected environment, the other Ancients could hear too. For in those moments of clarity, their minds became one. As they once had been, and were meant to be forever.

They were all created as one, and, thus, the Master had no name of its own. They all shared the one—Sariel—just as they shared one nature and one purpose. Their emotions and thought were naturally connected, in exactly the way the Master connected with the brood it was fostering, and all that would spring forth after that. The bond between the Ancients could be blocked but could never be broken. Their instincts and thoughts naturally yearned for connection.

In order to succeed, the Master had to subvert such an occurrence.

FALLEN LEAVES

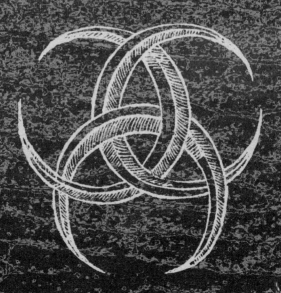

The Sewer

When Vasiliy regained consciousness, he found himself half-submerged in dirty water. All around him, ruptured pipes vomited gallons upon gallons of sewage water into the growing pool beneath him. Fet tried to get up, but leaned on his bad arm and groaned. He remembered what had happened: the explosion, the *strigoi*. The air was thick with the disturbing aroma of cooked flesh, mixed with toxic fumes. Somewhere in the distance—above him? beneath him?—he heard sirens and the squelch of police radios. Ahead, the faint glow of fire outlined a distant duct mouth.

His injured leg was submerged, still bleeding, adding to the murkiness of the water. His ears were still ringing, or, rather, just one. Fet raised his hand to it, and crusted blood flaked off into his fingers. He feared he had a blown eardrum.

He had no idea of where he was, or how he could get out, but the blast must have propelled him quite a way, and now, all around him, he found a little bit of free space.

He turned and located a loose grate near his flank. Rusty steel, rotten screws, rattling to his touch. He pried it loose a bit—and already he could feel a rush of fresh air. He was close to freedom, but his fingers were not enough to pry open the grate.

He felt around for something to use as a lever. He located a twisted length of steel—and then, lying facedown, the charred body of the *strigoi*.

As he looked at the burned remains, a moment of panic struck Fet. The blood worms. Had they seeped out of their host and blindly sought another body in this dank hole? If so, then . . . were they already in him? The wound in his leg? Would he feel any different if he was infected?

Then, the body moved.

It twitched.

Ever so slightly.

It was still functioning. Still alive—as alive as a vampire can be.

That was the reason the worms had not seeped out.

It stirred and sat up out of the water. Its back was charred, but not its front. Something was wrong with its eyes, and Fet knew in a moment that it no longer could see. It moved with sloppy determination, many of its bones fully dislocated yet its musculature still intact. Its jaw was no longer in place, ripped away by the blast, such that its stinger waved loosely in the air, like a tentacle.

The being splayed itself aggressively, a blind predator ready to charge. But Fet was transfixed by the sight of the exposed stinger. This was the first time he could see it completely. It was attached at two points, both at the base of the throat and at the back portion of the palate. The root was engorged and had a rippling, muscular structure. At the back of the throat, a sphincter-like hole gaped open in demand for food. Vasiliy thought he had seen a similar structure before—but where?

In the gloomy half-light, Fet felt around, looking for his nail gun. The creature's head turned to the water sounds, trying to orient itself. Fet was about to give up when he stumbled upon the nail gun—completely submerged in the water. *Damn*, he thought, trying to control his anger.

But the thing had locked on him, somehow—and charged. Fet moved as fast as he could, but now the creature, blindly adapted to the shape of the duct around it and its damaged limbs, instinctively found its footing, moving with uncanny coordination.

Fet raised the gun and hoped for luck. He pulled back on the trigger—twice—and found he was out of ammo. He had emptied the entire payload before being knocked out, and now was left with an empty industrial tool in his hand.

The thing was on top of him in a matter of seconds, tackling Fet, pushing him down.

Fet had its entire weight on top of him. What was left of its mouth trembled as the stinger recoiled, ready to shoot.

Reflexively, Vasiliy grabbed the stinger as he would a rabid rat. He pulled on it, bending it free of the structure of the thing's open throat. The thing squirmed and yelped, its dislocated arms unable to fight Fet's grip. The stinger was like a heavily muscled snake, slimy and squirming, bucking, trying to get loose. But now Vasiliy was angry. The harder the thing pulled back, the stronger Fet pulled forward. He would not give up his tight grip, his good arm pulling with all his might.

And Fet's might was immense.

In one final yank, Vasiliy overpowered the *strigoi* and ripped the stinger and part of the glandular structure and trachea from the thing's neck.

The entity squirmed in his hand, moving like an independent animal, even as the host body twitched spasmodically, falling back.

One thick blood worm emerged from the writhing mess, crawling quickly over Fet's fist. It slithered past his wrist and, all at once, began boring into his arm. It was drilling straight for the forearm veins, and Fet tossed away the stinger structure, watching this parasite invade his arm. It was halfway in when Vasiliy grabbed it by its visible, wriggling end, and yanked. He tore it back out, howling in pain and disgust. Again, reflex took over and he snapped the revolting parasite in two.

In his hands, before his eyes, the two halves

regenerated themselves—as if by magic—into complete parasites again.

Fet tossed them away. He saw, exiting the vampire's body, dozens of worms oozing out, slithering toward him through the fetid water.

His length of twisted steel gone, Fet said fuck it, ripping at the grate with his bare hands, pumped with adrenaline, tearing it loose and grabbing his empty nail gun as he jumped out of the duct and rushed to freedom.

The Silver Angel

HE LIVED ALONE in a tenement building in Jersey City, two blocks from Journal Square. One of the few neighborhoods that had not become gentrified. So many yuppies had taken over the rest—and where do they come from? How come they never end?

He climbed the steps to his fourth-floor apartment, his right knee creaking—literally creaking with every step—a squeak of pain jolting his body again and again.

His name was Angel Guzman Hurtado and he used to be big. He still was big, physically, but at age sixty-five his rebuilt knee hurt all the time and his body fat—what his American doctor called his BMI and what any Mexican would call *panza*—had overtaken his otherwise powerful figure. He sagged where he used to be taut, and he was taut where he had once been flexible— but big? Angel was always big. Both as a man and as a star—or at least what resembled it in his past life.

Angel had been a wrestler—*the* Wrestler back in Mexico City. El Angel de Plata. The Silver Angel.

He had begun his career in the 1960s as a *rudo* wrestler (one of the "bad guys"), but soon found himself embraced, with his trademark silver mask, by the adoring public, and so adjusted his style and altered his persona into a *tecnico*, one of the "good guys." Through the years he fashioned himself into an industry: comic books, *fotonovelas* (corny photo-illustrated magazines narrating his strange and often ridiculous exploits), films, and TV spots. He opened two gyms and bought half a dozen tenements throughout Mexico City, becoming, in his own right, a superhero of sorts. His films spanned all genres: western, horror, sci-fi, secret agent—many times within the same feature. He took on amphibian creatures as well as Soviet spies with equal aplomb in badly choreographed scenes full of library sound effects—always ending with his trademark knockout blow known as the "Angel Kiss."

But it was with vampires that he discovered his true niche. The silver-masked marvel battled every form of vampire: male, female, thin, fat—and, occasionally, even nude, for alternate versions exhibited only overseas.

But the eventual fall equaled the height of his climb. The more he expanded his brand empire, the more infrequently he trained, and wrestling became a nuisance he needed to put up with.

When his movies were box-office hits and his popularity still high, he performed wrestling exhibitions only once or twice a year. His movie *Angel vs. The Return of the Vampires* (a title that made no syntactic sense, and yet encapsulated his film oeuvre perfectly) found new life in repeated TV airings, and Angel felt compelled by fading fame to produce a cinematic rematch with those caped, fanged creatures that had given him so much.

And so it came to pass that one fine morning he found himself face-to-face with a group of young wrestlers made up as vampires in cheap greasepaint and rubber teeth. Angel himself walked them through a change in fight choreography that would have him wrapped three hours early—his focus less on the film at hand than on enjoying an afternoon martini back at the Intercontinental Hotel.

In the scene, one of the vampires would nearly unmask Angel until he miraculously freed himself with an open-palm blow, his trademark "Angel Kiss."

But as the scene progressed, filmed amid sweaty technicians at a stifling stage in Churubusco Studios, the younger vampire thespian, perhaps enraptured by the glory of his cinematic debut, applied a bit more force than necessary to their skirmish, and threw the middle-aged wrestler down. As they fell, the vampire adversary landed, both awkwardly and tragically, on his venerable master's leg.

Angel's knee snapped with a moist, loud crack,

bending into an almost perfect *L*—the wrestler's anguished scream muffled by his halfway torn silver mask.

He awoke hours later in a private room at one of Mexico's best hospitals, surrounded by flowers, serenaded by well-wishers shouting from the street below.

But his leg. It was shattered. Irreparably.

The good doctor explained this to him with genial forthrightness, a man with whom Angel had shared a few afternoons of craps at the country club across from the film studios.

In the months and years that followed, Angel spent a great deal of his fortune trying to repair his broken limb—in hopes of mending his fractured career and recovering his technique—but his skin hardened from the multiple scars crisscrossing the knee, and his bones refused to heal properly.

In a final humiliation, a newspaper revealed his identity to the public, and, without the ambiguity and the mystery of the silver mask, Angel the common man became too pitied to be adored.

The rest happened quickly. As his investments faltered, he worked as a trainer, then bodyguard, then as a bouncer, but his pride remained, and soon he found himself a burly old guy who scared no one. Fifteen years ago, he followed a woman to New York City and overstayed his visa. Now—like most people who end up in tenements—he had no clear idea how he had gotten here, only that he was indeed here, a resident in a building

quite similar to one of six he used to own outright.

But thinking of the past was dangerous and
painful.

Evenings, he worked as the dishwasher at the
Tandoori Palace downstairs, just next door. He
was able to stand for hours on busy nights by
wrapping lengths of duct tape around two broad
splints on either side of his knee, beneath his
trousers. And there were many busy nights. Now
and then, he cleaned the toilets and swept the
sidewalks, giving the Guptas enough reason to
keep him around. He had fallen to the bottom
of this caste system—so low that now his most
valuable possession was anonymity. No one had
to know who he once was. In a way, he was wearing a mask again.

For the past two evenings, the Tandoori Palace
had remained closed—as had the grocery store
next door, the other half of the neo-Bengali em-
porium the Guptas owned. No word from them,
and no sign of their presence, no answer at their
phone. Angel started to worry—no, not about
them, truthfully, but about his income. The radio
talked of quarantine, which was good for health
but very bad for business. Had the Guptas fled
the city? Perhaps they had gotten caught in some
of the violence that had cropped up? In all this
chaos, how would he know if they had been shot?

Three months before, they had sent him out
to make duplicates of the keys to both places. He
had made triplicates—he didn't know what had

possessed him, certainly no dark impulse on his part but only a lesson learned in life: to be prepared for anything.

Tonight, he decided, he would take a look. He needed to know. Just before dusk, Angel hauled himself down to the Guptas' store. The street was quiet except for a dog, a black husky he had never seen in the neighborhood, barking at him from across the sidewalk—though something stopped the dog from crossing the street.

The Guptas' store had once been called The Taj Mahal, but now, after generations of graffiti and pamphlet removal, the painted logo had worn away so that only the rosy illustration of the Indian Wonder of the World remained. Strangely, it exhibited too many minarets.

Now, someone had defaced the logo even further, spray-painting a cryptic design of lines and dots in fluorescent orange. The design, cryptic though it was, was fresh. The paint still glistened, a few threads of it slowly dripping at the corners.

Vandals. Here. Yet the locks were in place, the door undamaged.

Angel turned the key. When both bolts slid free, he limped inside.

Everything was silent. The power had been cut, and so the refrigerator was off, all the meats and fish inside gone to waste. Light from the last of the sunset filtered in through the steel shutters over the windows, like an orange-gold mist. Deeper inside, the store was dark. Angel had brought two busted cell phones with him. The call functions did not work, but the screens and batteries still did, and he found that—thanks to a picture of his white wall he snapped during daylight—the screens made excellent lights for hanging on his belt or even strapped to his head for close work.

The store was in absolute disarray. Rice and lentils covered the floor, spilled from several overturned containers. The Guptas would never have allowed this.

Something, Angel knew, was deeply wrong.

Above all else was the stench of ammonia. Not the eye-watering odor of the off-the-shelf cleaner kind he used to clean the toilets, but something more foul. Not pure like a chemical, but messy and organic. His phone illuminated several streaking trails of orange-tinged fluid along the floor, sticky and still wet. They led to the cellar door.

The basement beneath the store communicated with the restaurant and, ultimately, with the belowground floors of his tenement building.

Angel put a shoulder to the Guptas' office door. He knew they kept an old handgun inside the desk. He found it, the weapon feeling heavy and oily, not at all like the shiny prop guns he used to wave around. He tucked one of the phones into his tight belt and returned to the cellar door.

With his leg hurting more than ever, the old wrestler started down the slick steps. At the bottom, a door. This one had been broken, Angel saw—but from the inside. Someone had broken in from the cellar up to the store.

Beyond the storeroom, Angel heard a hissing sound, evenly measured and prolonged. He went in with both the gun and his phone out.

Another design defaced the wall. It resembled a bloom of six petals, or perhaps an inkblot: the center done in gold, the petals painted black. The paint still glistened, and he ran his light over all of it—maybe a bug, not a flower—before squeezing through the doorway into the next room.

The ceiling was low, spaced with wooden beams for support. Angel knew the layout well. One passage led to a narrow stairway to the sidewalk, where they received food shipments three times a week. The other burrowed through to his tenement building. He started ahead toward his building when the toe of his shoe hit something.

He aimed his phone light down onto the floor. At first he did not understand it. A person, sleeping. Then another. And two more near the stack of chairs.

They weren't sleeping, because he didn't hear any snoring or deep breathing, and yet they weren't dead, because he didn't smell death.

At that very moment, outside, the last of the sun's direct rays disappeared from the East Coast sky. Night was upon the city, and newly turned vampires, those in their first days, responded very literally to the cosmic edict of sundown and sunup.

The slumbering vampires began to stir. Angel had stumbled unwittingly into a vast nest of undead. He did not need to wait to see their faces to know that this—people rising en masse from the floor of a darkened cellar—was not anything he wanted to be part of, nor indeed present for.

He moved to the narrow space in the wall

toward the burrow to his building—one he had seen both ends of but never had the occasion to cross—only to see more figures beginning to rise, blocking his way.

He did not yell or give any warning. He fired the weapon, but was not prepared for the intensity of light and sound inside that constricted space.

Nor were his targets, who appeared more affected by the reports and the bright flash of flame than they were by the lead rounds that pierced their bodies. He fired three more times, achieving the same effect, and then twice behind him, sensing the others' approach.

The gun clicked empty.

He threw it down. Only one option remained. An old door he had never opened—because he had never been able to, a door with no knob or handle, stuck within a compressed wooden frame surrounded by rock wall.

Angel pretended it was a prop door. Told himself it was a breakaway piece of balsa wood. He had to. He gripped the phone in his fist and lowered his shoulder and ran at it full-force.

The old wood scraped away from its frame, dislodging dust and dirt as the lock cracked and it burst open. Angel and his balky leg stumbled through—nearly falling into a gang of punks on the other side.

The bangers raised guns and silver swords at him, staggered by his bulk, about to slay him.

"Madre Santisima!" exclaimed Angel. Holy Mother of God!

Gus, at the head of the pack, was about to run this vampire motherfucker through when he heard him speak—and speak Spanish. The words stopped Gus—and the vampire-hunting Sapphires behind him—just in time.

"Me lleva la chingada—que haces tu aca, muchachon?" said Gus. What the fuck are you doing here, big boy?

Angel said nothing, letting his facial expression do all the talking as he turned and pointed behind him.

"More bloodsuckers," said Gus, understanding. "That's what we're here for." He stared at the big man. There was something noble and familiar about him.

"Te conozco?" said Gus. Do I know you? To which the wrestler answered with a quick shrug, but no more words.

Alfonso Creem charged through the doorway, armed with a thick silver rapier with a bell-cup hilt to protect his hand from the blood worms. That protection was negated by the use of his other hand, bare except for a silver-knuckled multi-finger ring inscribed with fake diamonds spelling C-R-E-E-M.

He went after the vampires with furious chops and brutal blows. Gus was right behind him, a UV lamp in one hand, a silver sword in the other. More Sapphires followed close behind.

Never fight in a basement was a tenet of both street fighting and warfare, but it couldn't be avoided in a vamp hunt. Gus would have preferred to firebomb the place, if he could be guaranteed full mortality. But these vamps always seemed to have another way out.

There were more nesting vamps than they had bargained for, and the white blood spilled like sludgy, sour milk. Still, they cut and chopped their way through, and, when they were done, they returned to Angel, who remained standing on the other side of the broken door.

Angel was in a state of shock. He had recognized the Guptas among Creem's victims, and he couldn't get over their undead faces, and the creature howls they emitted when the Colombian hacked at their white-blooded throats.

These were the types of punks he used to slap around in his movies. *"Que chingados pasa?"* What is all this?

"The end of the world," said Gus. "Who are you?"

"I'm . . . I am nobody," Angel said, recovering. "I worked here." He pointed up at an angle. "Live there."

"Your entire building is infested, man."

"Infested? Are they really . . . ?"

"Vampires? You bet your ass."

Angel felt dizzy—disoriented—this couldn't be happening. Not to him. A whirl of emotions overtook him and amid them he was able to recognize one that had long ago deserted him.

It was excitement.

Creem was flexing his silver fist. "Leave him. These freaks are waking up all over the place, and I still got some more killing in me."

"What do you say?" asked Gus, turning back to

his fellow countryman. "Nothing for you here."

"Look at that knee," said Creem. "No one's going to slow me up, get me turned into one of them stingers."

Gus pulled a small sword from the Sapphires' equipment bag and handed it to Angel. "This is his building. Let's see if he can earn his keep."

As though some sort of psychic alarm had been sounded, the vampire residents of Angel's building were ready for battle. The undead emerged from every doorway, climbing effortlessly through obstacles and staircases.

During a stairway battle, Angel saw a neighbor of his, a seventy-three-year-old woman with a walker, use the banister as a jumping point to traverse the stairwell between floors. She and others moved with the stupefying grace of primates.

In his movies, the enemy announced itself with a glower, and accommodated the hero by moving slowly for the kill. Angel didn't exactly "earn his keep," though his brute strength did give him certain advantages. His wrestling knowledge came back to him in close combat situations, despite his limited mobility. And he felt like an action hero once again.

Like evil spirits, the undead kept coming. As though summoned from the surrounding buildings, wave after wave of pale, slithery-tongued creatures swarmed up from the lower floors, and the tenement walls ran white. They fought them the way firemen fight fires, pushing back, tamping out flare-ups, and attacking hot spots. They functioned as a stone-cold execution squad, and Angel would later be amazed to learn that this was their inaugural nighttime assault. Two of the Colombians were stung, lost to the scourge—and yet when they were done, the punks only seemed to want more.

Compared to this, they said, daylight hunting was a breeze.

Once they had stemmed the tide, one of the Colombians found a carton of smokes and they all lit up. Angel hadn't smoked in years, but the taste and the smell blocked out the stench of the dead things. Gus watched the smoke dissipate and offered up a silent prayer for the departed.

"There is a man," said Gus. "An old pawnbroker over in Manhattan. He was the first to clue me to these vamps. Saved my soul."

"No chance," said Creem. "Why go all the way across the river when there is killing galore here?"

"You meet this guy, you'll understand why."

"How do you know he's still kickin' it?"

"I sure hope he is. We're going over the bridge at first light."

Angel took a minute then to return to his apartment for the last time. His knee ached as he looked around: unwashed clothes heaped in the corner, dirty dishes in his sink, the general squalor of the place. He had never taken any pride in his living condition—and it shamed him now. Perhaps, he sensed, he knew all the time that he was destined for something better—something he could never have foreseen—and he was just waiting for the call.

He threw some extra clothes into a grocery bag, including his knee brace, and then lastly—almost ashamedly, because taking it was like admitting it was his most cherished possession, all he had left of who he once was—he grabbed the silver mask.

He folded the mask into his jacket pocket and, with it next to his heart, he realized that, for the first time in decades, he felt good about himself.

The Flatlands

EPH FINISHED TENDING to Vasiliy's injuries, giving particular attention to cleaning out the worm hole in his forearm. The rat-catcher had sustained a great deal of damage, but none of it permanent, except maybe the hearing loss and ringing in his right ear. The metal shard came out of his leg and he hobbled on it but did not complain. He was still standing. Eph admired that, and felt a bit like an Ivy League momma's boy by his side. For all his education and scholarly achievements, Eph felt infinitely less useful to the cause than Fet.

But that would soon change.

The exterminator opened his poison closet, showing Setrakian his bait packs and traps, his halothane bottles and toxic blue kibble. Rats, he explained, lacked the biological mechanism for vomiting. The main function of emesis is to purge a body of toxic substances, which was why rats were particularly susceptible to poisoning. Why they had evolved and developed other traits to compensate for this. One was that they could ingest just about anything, including nonfood materials such as clay or concrete, which helped to dilute a toxin's effect on the rat's body until they could get rid of the poison as waste. The other was the rats' intelligence, their complex food-avoidance strategies that aided in their survival.

"Funny thing," said Fet, "is that when I ripped out that thing's throat, and got a good look in there?"

"Yes?" said Setrakian.

"The way it looked to me, I'd bet dollars to doughnuts they can't puke either."

Setrakian nodded, thinking on that. "I believe you are correct," he said. "May I ask, what is the chemical makeup of these rodenticides?"

"Depends," said Fet. "These use thallium sulfate, a heavy metal salt that attacks the liver, brain, and muscle. Odorless, colorless, and highly toxic. These over here use a common mammalian blood-thinner."

"Mammalian? What, something like Coumadin?"

"No, not something like. Exactly like."

Setrakian looked at the bottle. "So I myself have been taking rat poison for some years now."

"Yep. You and millions of other people."

"And this does what?"

"Same thing it would do to you if you took too much of it. The anticoagulant leads to internal hemorrhaging. Rats bleed out. It's not pretty."

In picking up the bottle to examine its label, Setrakian noticed something on the shelf behind it. "I do not wish to alarm you, Vasiliy. But aren't these mouse droppings?"

Fet pushed his way in for a closer look. "Motherfucker!" he said. "How can this be?"

"A minor infestation, I'm sure," said Setrakian.

"Minor, major, what does it matter? This is supposed to be Fort Knox!" Fet knocked over a few bottles, trying to see better. "This is like vampires breaking into a silver mine."

While Fet was obsessively searching the back of the closet for more evidence, Eph watched Setrakian slip one of the bottles inside his coat pocket.

Eph followed Setrakian away from the closet, catching him alone. "What are you going to do with that?" he said.

Setrakian showed no guilt at having been discovered. The old man's cheeks were sunken, his flesh a pale shade of gray. "He said it is essentially blood thinner. With all the pharmacies being raided, I would not like to run out."

Eph studied the old man, trying to see the truth behind his lie.

Setrakian said, "Nora and Zack are ready for their journey to Vermont?"

"Just about. But not Vermont. Nora had a good point—it's Kelly's parents' place, she might be drawn to it. There's a girls' camp Nora knows, from growing up in Philadelphia. It's off-season now. Three cabins on a small island in the middle of a lake."

"Good," said Setrakian. "The water will keep them safe. How soon do you leave for the train station?"

"Soon," said Eph, checking his wristwatch. "We still have a little time."

"They could take a car. You do realize that we are out of the epicenter now. This neighborhood, with its lack of direct subway service and comparatively few apartment buildings conducive to rapid infestation, has yet to be totally colonized. We are not in a bad spot here."

Eph shook his head. "The train is the fastest and surest way out of this plague."

Setrakian said, "Fet told me about the off-duty policemen who came to the pawnshop. Who resorted to vigilantism once their families were safely away from the city. You have something similar in mind, I think."

Eph was stunned. Had the old man intuited his plan somehow? He was about to tell him when Nora entered carrying an open carton. "What is this stuff for?" she asked, setting it down near the raccoon cages. Inside were chemicals and trays. "You setting up a dark room?"

Setrakian turned from Eph. "There are certain silver emulsions that I want to test on blood worms. I am optimistic that a fine mist of silver, if possible to derive, synthesize, and direct, will be an effective weapon for mass killing of the creatures."

Nora said, "But how are you going to test it? Where are you going to get a blood worm?"

Setrakian lifted the lid off a Styrofoam cooler, revealing the jar containing his slowly pulsing vampire heart. "I will segment the worm powering this organ."

Eph said, "Isn't that dangerous?"

"Only if I make a mistake. I have segmented the parasites in the past. Each section regenerates a fully functioning worm."

"Yeah," said Fet, returning from the poison closet. "I've seen it."

Nora lifted out the jar, looking at the heart the old man had fed for more than thirty years, keeping it alive with his own blood. "Wow," she said. "It's like a symbol, isn't it?"

Setrakian looked at her with keen interest. "How do you mean?"

"This diseased heart kept in a jar. I don't know. I think it exemplifies that which will be our ultimate downfall."

Eph said, "Being what?"

Nora looked at him with an expression of both sadness and sympathy. "Love," she said.

"Ah," said Setrakian, his acknowledgment confirming her insight.

"The undead returning for their Dear Ones," Nora said. "Human love corrupted into vampiric need."

Setrakian said, "That may indeed be the most insidious evil of this plague. That is why you have to destroy Kelly."

Nora quickly agreed. "You must release her from the Master's grip. Release Zack. And, by extension, all of us."

Eph was shocked but knew all too well that she was right. "I know," he said.

"But it is not enough to know what is the correct course of action," said Setrakian. "You are being called upon to perform a deed that goes against every human instinct. And, in the act of releasing a loved one . . . you taste what it is to be turned. To go against everything you are. That act changes one forever."

Setrakian's words had power, and the others were silent. Then Zack—evidently tired of playing the handheld video game Eph had found for him, or perhaps the battery had finally given out—returned from the van, finding them gathered in conversation. "What's going on?"

"Nothing, young man—talking strategy," said Setrakian, taking a seat on one of the cartons, resting his legs. "Vasiliy and I have an appointment in Manhattan, so, with your father's permission, we will catch a ride with you back over the bridge."

Eph said, "What kind of appointment?"

"At Sotheby's, a preview of their next auction."

"I thought they weren't offering that item for preview."

"They are not," said Setrakian. "But we have to try. This is my absolute last chance. At the very least, it will give Vasiliy the opportunity to observe their security."

Zack looked at his dad and said, "Can't we do the James Bond security stuff instead of getting on a train?"

Eph said, "'Fraid not, little ninja. You gotta go."

Nora said, "But how will you all keep in touch and connect afterward?" She pulled out her phone. "This thing is just a camera now. They're toppling cell towers in every borough."

Setrakian said, "If worse comes to worst, we can always meet back here. Perhaps you should use the ground line to contact your mother, tell her we are on the way."

Nora left to do just that, and Fet went out to start the van. Then it was just Eph and Zack, the father with his arm around his son, facing the old man.

"You know, Zachary," said Setrakian, "in the camp I was telling you about, the conditions were so brutal that many times I wanted to grab a rock, a hammer, a shovel, and take down one, maybe two guards. I would have died with them, for certain—and yet, in the searing heat of the moment of choice, at least I would have accomplished *something*. At least my life—my death—would have meaning."

Setrakian never looked at Eph, only the boy, though Eph knew this speech was meant for him.

"That was how I thought. And every day I despised myself for not going through with it. Every moment of inaction feels like cowardice in the face of such inhuman oppression. Survival often feels like an indignity. But—and this is the lesson as I see it now, as an old man—sometimes the most difficult decision is to not martyr yourself for someone, but instead to choose to live *for* them. *Because* of them."

Only then did he look at Eph.

"I do hope you will take that to heart."

The Black Forest Solutions Facility

THE CUSTOM VAN in the middle of a three-vehicle motorcade pulled to a stop right outside the canopied entrance of the Black Forest Solutions meatpacking facility in Upstate New York.

Handlers from both the lead and trailing SUVs opened large black umbrellas as the rear van doors opened and an automatic ramp was lowered to the driveway.

A wheelchair was rolled out backward, its occupant immediately surrounded by the umbrellas and quickly shuttled inside.

The umbrellas did not come down until the chair reached a windowless expanse among the animal pens. The occupant of the wheelchair was a sun-shy figure wearing a burka-like habit.

Eldritch Palmer, watching the entrance from the side, made no attempt to greet the occupant, but instead awaited its unveiling. Palmer was supposed to be meeting with the Master, not one of its wretched Third Reich flunkies. But the Dark One was nowhere to be seen. Palmer realized then that he had not had an audience with the Master since its run-in with Setrakian.

A small, impolite smile curled the edges of Palmer's lips. Was he pleased that the disgraced professor had shown the Master some disgrace? No, not exactly. Palmer had zero affection for lost causes such as Abraham Setrakian. Still, as a man used to being president and CEO, Palmer didn't mind that the Master had been shown something in the way of humility.

He chastised himself then, admonishing himself to never let these thoughts enter his mind in the presence of the Dark One.

The Nazi removed his coverings layer by layer. Thomas Eichhorst, the Nazi who had once headed the Treblinka extermination camp, arose from the wheelchair, the black sun-coverings piled at his feet like so many sloughed layers of flesh. His face retained the arrogance of a camp commandant, though the decades had worn away the edges like a fine acid. His flesh was smooth as a mask of ivory. Unlike any other Eternal Palmer had ever met, Eichhorst insisted on wearing a suit and tie, maintaining the bearing of an undead gentleman.

Palmer's dislike for the Nazi had nothing whatsoever to do with his crimes against humanity. Palmer was in the midst of overseeing a genocide himself. Rather, his distaste for Eichhorst was borne out of envy. He resented Eichhorst's blessing of Eternity—the great gift of the Master— because he coveted it so.

Palmer then recalled his first introduction to the Master, a meeting facilitated by Eichhorst. This had followed three full decades of searching and researching, of exploring that seam where myth and legend met historical reality. Palmer finally tracked down the Ancients themselves, and finagled an introduction. They turned down his request to join their Eternal clan, refusing him flatly, even though Palmer knew they had accepted into their rare breed men whose net worth was significantly lower than his. Their unqualified scorn, after so many years of hope, was a humiliation that Eldritch Palmer simply could not bear. It meant his mortality and the surrender of all that he had accomplished in this pre-life. Ashes to ashes and dust to dust: that was fine for the masses, but for Palmer, only immortality would do. The corruption of his body—which had never been a friend to him—was but a small price to pay.

And so commenced another decade of searching—but this time, in pursuit of the legend of the rogue Ancient, the seventh immortal, whose power was said to rival any of the others. This journey brought Palmer to the craven Eichhorst, who arranged the summit.

It occurred inside the Zone of Alienation surrounding the Chernobyl Nuclear Power Plant in the Ukraine, a little more than a decade after the 1986 reactor disaster. Palmer had to enter the Zone without his usual motorcade support (his unmarked ambulance and security detail), the reason being that moving vehicles kick up radioactive dust, laced with cesium-137, so you don't want to follow any other moving vehicles. So Mr. Fitzwilliam—Palmer's bodyguard and medic—drove him alone, and drove fast.

Their meeting took place after nightfall, of course, in one of the so-called black villages surrounding the plant: evacuated settlements that dotted the most blighted ten-square-kilometer area of the planet.

Pripyat, the largest of these settlements, had been founded in 1970 to house plant workers, its population having grown to fifty thousand at the time of the accident and radiation exposure. The city was fully evacuated three days later. A carnival had been built in a large downtown lot, set to open on May 1, 1986: five days after the disaster, two days after the city was emptied forever.

Palmer met the Master at the foot of the never-operated Ferris wheel, sitting as still as a giant stopped clock. It was there that a deal was struck, and the Ten-year Plan set into motion—with the Earth's occultation designated as the time of the crossing.

In return, Palmer was promised his Eternity, and a seat at the right hand of the Master. Not as one of his errand-boy acolytes but as a partner in apocalypse, pending his delivery of the human race as promised.

Before the meeting ended, the Master grasped Palmer by the arm and ran up the side of the giant Ferris wheel. At the top, the terrified Palmer was shown Chernobyl, the red beacon of the #4 reactor in the distance, pulsing steadily atop the sarcophagus of lead and steel, sealing in one hundred tons of labile uranium.

And now here he was, ten years on, Palmer at the verge of delivering everything he had pledged to the Master on that dark night in a diseased land. The plague was spreading faster every hour now, throughout the country and across the globe—and still he was being made to bear the indignity of this vampire bureaucrat.

Eichhorst's expertise was in the construction of animal pens and the coordination of maximally efficient abattoirs. Palmer had financed the "refurbishing" of dozens of meat plants nationwide, all of them redesigned according to Eichhorst's exact specifications.

I trust everything is in order, said Eichhorst.

"Naturally," said Palmer, barely able to mask his distaste for the creature. "What I want to know is, when will the Master uphold his end of the bargain?"

In due time. All in due time.

"My time is due *now*," said Palmer. "You know the condition of my health. You know that I have fulfilled every promise, that I have met every deadline, that I have served your Master faithfully and completely. Now the hour grows late. I am due some consideration."

The Dark Lord sees everything and forgets nothing.

"I will remind you of his—and your—unfinished business with Setrakian, your former pet prisoner."

His resistance is doomed.

"Agreed, of course. And yet his operations and his diligence do pose a threat to some individuals. Including yourself. And me."

Eichhorst was silent a moment, as though conceding his agreement.

The Master will settle his affairs with the Juden in a matter of hours. Now—I have not fed for some time, and I was promised a fresh meal.

Palmer hid a frown of disgust. How quickly his human revulsion would turn to hunger, to need. How soon he would look back upon his naiveté here the way an adult looks back upon the needs of a child. "Everything has been arranged."

Eichhorst motioned to one of his handlers who stepped away into one of the larger pens. Palmer heard whimpering and checked his watch, wanting to be done with this.

Eichhorst's handler returned holding, by the back of his neck, much as a farmer might lift up a piglet, a boy of no more than eleven years of age. Blindfolded and shivering, the boy pawed at the air before him, kicking, trying to see beneath the cloth covering his eyes.

Eichhorst turned his head at the smell of his victim, his chin tipped in a gesture of appreciation.

Palmer observed the Nazi and wondered for a moment what it would feel like, after the pain of the turning. What will it mean to exist as a creature who feeds on man?

Palmer turned and signaled to Mr. Fitzwilliam to start the car. "I will leave you to eat in peace," he said, and left the vampire to its meal.

International Space Station

TWO HUNDRED AND twenty miles above Earth, the concepts of day and night had little meaning. Orbiting the planet once every hour and a half provided all the dawns and sunsets a person could handle.

Astronaut Thalia Charles gently snored inside a sleeping bag strapped to the wall. The American flight engineer was entering her 466th day in Low Earth orbit, with only 6 more to go before the space shuttle docking that was to be her ride back home.

Mission Control set their sleep schedules, and today was to be an "early" day, readying the ISS to receive *Endeavor* and the next research facility module it carried. She heard the voice summoning her, and spent a pleasant few seconds transforming from sleep to wakefulness. The floating sensation of dreaming is a constant in zero gravity. She wondered how her head would react to a pillow upon her return. What it would be like to come under the benevolent dictatorship of Earth's gravity once again.

She removed her eye mask and neck pad, tucking each inside the sleeping bag before loosening the straps and wriggling out. She undid her elastic and shook out her long, black hair, combing it apart with her fingers, then turning a half-somersault to regather it and wind the elastic back around in a double loop.

The voice of Mission Control from Houston's Johnson Space Center called her to the laptop in the Unity module for a teleconference uplink. This was unusual but not, in itself, a cause for alarm. Bandwidth in space is in high demand, and very carefully allocated. She wondered if there hadn't been another orbital collision of space junk, its debris rocketed through orbit with the force of a shotgun blast. She disdained having to take shelter inside the attached *Soyuz-TMA* spacecraft, as a precaution. The *Soyuz* was their emergency escape from the ISS. A similar threat had occurred two months ago, necessitating an eight-day stay inside its bell-shaped crew module. Space-junk hazards posed the greatest threat to the viability of the ISS, and to the psychological well-being of its crew.

The news, as she found out, was even worse.

"We're scrapping the *Endeavor* launch for now," said Mission Control head Nicole Fairley.

"Scrapping? You mean postponing?" said Thalia, trying not to betray too much disappointment.

"Postponing indefinitely. There's a lot going on down here. Some troubling developments. We need to wait this out."

"What? The thrusters again?"

"No, nothing mechanical. *Endeavor* is sound. This is not a technical problem."

"Okay . . ."

"To be honest, I don't know what this is. You may have noticed you haven't received any news updates these past few days."

There was no direct Internet access in space. Astronauts received data, video, and e-mail through a Kû-band data link. "Do we have another virus?" All the laptops on the ISS operated on a wireless intranet, segregated from the mainframe.

"Not a computer virus, no."

Thalia gripped the handlebar to hold herself still in front of the screen. "Okay. I'm going to stop asking questions now and just listen."

"We are in the midst of a rather mystifying global pandemic. It apparently started in Manhattan and has been popping up in various cities and spreading ever since. Concurrently, and apparently in direct relation, there have been a large number of disappearances reported. At first, these vanishings were attributed to sick people staying home from work, people seeking medical attention. Now there are riots. I'm talking entire blocks of New York City. The violence has spread across state lines. The first report of attacks in London came four days ago, then at Narita Airport in Japan. Each country has been guarding its flank and its international profile, trying to avoid a meltdown of travel and commerce, which—as I understand it—is, in fact, exactly what each country *should* be seeking. The World Health Organization held a press conference yesterday in Berlin. Half of its members were absent. They officially moved the pandemic from a phase five to a phase-six alert."

Thalia couldn't believe it. "Is it the eclipse?" she said.

"What's that?"

"The occultation. When I watched it from up

here . . . the great black blot that was the shadow of the moon, spreading over the northeastern U.S. like a dead spot . . . I guess I had this . . . I had a premonition of sorts."

"Well—it does seem to have started around then."

"It was just the way it looked. So ominous."

"We have had a few major incidents here in Houston, and more in Austin and Dallas. Mission Control is operating at about seventy percent manpower now, our numbers shrinking every day. With operation personnel levels unreliable, we have no choice but to push back the launch at this time."

"Okay. I understand."

"The Russian transport that went up two months ago left you plenty of food and batteries, enough to last up to a year if rationing becomes necessary."

"A *year*?" said Thalia, more forcefully than she would have liked.

"Just thinking worst-case. Hopefully things get back under control here and we can get you back maybe two or three weeks out."

"Great. So until then, more freeze-dried borscht."

"This same message is being relayed to Commander Demidov and Engineer Maigny by their respective agencies. We are aware of your disappointment, Thalia."

"I haven't received any e-mail from my husband in a few days. Have you been holding those back as well?"

"No, we haven't. A few days, you say?"

Thalia nodded. She pictured Billy as she always did, working inside the kitchen of their home in West Hartford, dishrag over his shoulder, cooking up some ambitious feast over the stove. "Contact him for me, will you? He'll want to know about the postponement."

"We did attempt to contact him. No answer. Either at your house, or his restaurant."

Thalia swallowed hard. She worked quickly to regain her composure.

He's fine, she thought. *I'm the one orbiting the planet in a spaceship. He's down there, both feet on the ground. He's fine.*

She showed Mission Control only confidence and fortitude, but she had never felt so far away from her husband as at that moment.

Knickerbocker Loans and Curios, East 118th Street, Spanish Harlem

THE BLOCK WAS already burning when Gus arrived with the Sapphires and Angel.

They saw smoke from the bridge on the way over: thick and black, rising in various spots uptown and down, Harlem and the Lower East Side and points between. As though the city had seen a coordinated military attack.

The morning sun was overhead, the city quiet. They shot up Riverside Drive, weaving around abandoned vehicles. Seeing smoke rising from city blocks was like watching a person bleed. Gus felt alternately helpless and anxious—the city was falling to shit all around him, and time was of the essence.

Creem and the other Jersey punks looked upon Manhattan burning with a kind of satisfaction. To them it was like watching a disaster movie. But to Gus, this was like watching his turf going up in flames.

The block they were headed to was the epicenter of the biggest uptown blaze: all the streets surrounding the pawnshop were blacked out by the thick veil of smoke, turning day into a strange, storm-like night.

"Those motherfuckers," said Gus. "They blocked out the sun."

The entire side of the street raged in flames—except the pawnshop on the corner. Its large front windows were shattered, security grates pulled off the building overhang and lying twisted on the sidewalk.

The rest of the city was quieter than a cold Christmas morning, but this block—the 118th Street intersection—was, at that dark daylight hour, teeming with vamps laying siege to the pawnshop.

They were after the old man.

Inside the apartment above the shop, Gabriel Bolivar moved from room to room. Silver-backed mirrors covered the walls instead of pictures, as though some strange spell had converted artwork into glass. The former rock star's blurry reflection moved with him from room to room in his search for the old man Setrakian and his accomplices.

Bolivar stopped in the room the mother of the boy had tried to enter—the wall boarded behind an iron cage.

No one.

It looked as though they had cleared out. Bolivar wished the mother had accompanied them here. Her blood link to the boy would have proved valuable. But the Master had tasked Bolivar, and its will would be done.

The job of bloodhound instead fell to the feelers, the newly turned blind children. Bolivar came out to the kitchen to see one there, a boy with fully black eyes, crouching down on all fours. He was "looking" out the window toward the street, using his extrasensory perception.

The basement? said Bolivar.

No one, said the boy.

But Bolivar needed to see it for himself, needed to be sure, moving past him to the stairs. Bolivar rode the spiral railing down on his hands and bare feet, down one floor to the street level, where the other feelers had retreated to the shop—then continuing his descent to the basement and a locked door.

Bolivar's soldiers were already there, in answer to his telepathic command. They tore at the locked door with powerful, oversize hands, digging into the iron-bolted frame with the hardened nails of their talon-like middle fingers until they gained purchase, then joined forces to rip the door back from its frame.

The first few to enter tripped the ultraviolet lamps surrounding the interior of the doorway, the electric indigo rays cooking their virus-rich bodies, the vampires dissipating with screams and clouds of dust. The rest were repulsed by the light, pushed backward against the spiral staircase, shading their eyes. They were unable to see through the doorway.

Bolivar was the first to haul himself hand over hand up the staircase, ahead of the crush. The old man still could be inside there.

Bolivar had to find another way in.

He noticed then the feelers tensed on the floor, facing the smashed windows and the street beyond, like pointer dogs responding to a scent. The first among them—a girl in soiled briefs and an undershirt—snarled and then leaped through the jagged shards of glass to the street.

The little girl came right at Angel, loping on all fours with fawn-like grace. The old wrestler backed up into the street, wanting no part of her, but she had locked in on the biggest target and was set on taking him down. She sprang up from the road, black-eyed, open-mouthed—and Angel reverted into wrestler mode, handling her as though she were a challenger throwing herself at him from the top turnbuckle. He applied the Angel Kiss, his open-palm blow smacking the girl out of the air in mid-leap, sending her lithe little body flying a good dozen yards away, tumbling to the road.

Angel recoiled immediately. One of the great disappointments of his life was not knowing any of the children he had sired. She was a vampire, but she looked so human—a child, still—and he started toward her with his bare hand outstretched. She turned and hissed, her blind eyes like two black bird's eggs, her stinger darting out at him, maybe three feet in length, considerably shorter than an adult vampire's. The tip flailed before his eyes like a devil's tail, and Angel was transfixed.

Gus intervened quickly, finishing her with a hard swipe of his sword that scored the surface of the road, scraping up sparks.

This slaying sent the other vamps into an attack frenzy. A brutal battle, Gus and the Sapphires outnumbered at first three to one, then four to one as vamps fled from the pawnshop and emerged from the basements of the adjacent buildings burning along the street. Either they had been psychically summoned into battle, or simply heard the ringing dinner bell. Destroy one, and two more came at you.

Then a shotgun blast exploded near Gus and a marauding vamp was cut in two. He turned to see Mr. Quinlan, the Ancients' chief hunter, picking off rioting white-bloods with military precision. He must have come up from underneath like these others. Unless he had been shadowing Gus and the Sapphires the entire time, from the darkness of the underground.

Gus noticed, in that moment—his senses heightened by the adrenaline of battle—that no blood worms coursed beneath the surface of Quinlan's translucent skin. All the old ones, including the other hunters, crawled with worms, and yet his nearly iridescent flesh was as still and smooth as skin on a pudding.

But the fight was on, and the revelation passed in an instant. Mr. Quinlan's killing cleared some much-needed space, and the Sapphires, no longer in danger of being surrounded, moved the fight from the middle of the street toward the pawnshop. The children waited, on all fours, on the periphery of the battle, like wolf cubs awaiting a weakened deer to kill. Quinlan sent one blast in their direction, the blind creatures scattering with a high-pitched squeal as he reloaded.

Angel snapped a vampire's neck with a sharp twist of his hands, and then, in a single, swift move, rare for a man his age—and girth—he turned and used his massive elbow to crack the skull of another one against the wall.

Gus saw his chance, and broke away from the melee, running inside with his sword in search of the old man. The shop was empty, so he ran up the stairs, into an old, prewar apartment.

The many mirrors told him he was in the right place—but no old man.

He met two female vamps on the way back down, introducing them to the heel of his boot before running them through with silver. Their shrieks adrenalized him as he jumped over their bodies, avoiding the white blood oozing down the steps.

The stairs continued belowground, but he had to return to his *compadres* fighting for their lives and their souls beneath the smoke-blotted sky.

Before exiting, he noticed a section of busted wall near the stairs, exposing old copper water pipes running vertically. He set his sword down on a display case of brooches and cameos, finding a Chuck Knoblauch–autographed Louisville Slugger baseball bat with a $39.99 price tag. He hacked away at the old wallboard, smashing it open until he located the gas line. An old cast-iron pipe. Three good hacks with the bat, and it separated at a coupling—fortunately, without producing any sparks.

The smell of natural gas filled the room, escaping from the ruptured pipe not with a cool hiss but with a hoarse roar.

The feelers swarmed around Bolivar, who felt their distress.

This fighter with the shotgun. He was not human. He was vampire.

But he was different.

The feelers could not read him. Even if he were of a different clan—and, clearly, he was—they should have been able to impart some knowledge of him to Bolivar, so long as he was of the worm.

Bolivar was mystified by this strange presence, and made to attack. But the feelers, reading his intent, leaped into his path. He tried to pull them off, but their dogged insistence was strange enough to merit his attention.

Something was about to happen, and he needed to take heed.

Gus reclaimed his sword and slashed his way out through another vamp—this one dressed in doctor's scrubs—on his way outside and into the next building. There, he ripped away a burning section of windowsill, running with the flaming plank back into battle. He drove it, sharp point–down, into the back of a slain vamp, so that the wood stood like a torch.

"Creem!" he called, needing the silver-blinged killer to cover him as he went into the gear bag for the crossbow. He rummaged for a silver bolt, finding one. Gus tore off a piece of the downed vamp's shirt, wrapping it around the bolt head and tying it tight, then loading the bolt into the cross, dipping the wrapping into the flames, and raising the crossbow toward the store.

A vamp wearing bloody gym clothes came wilding at Gus, and Quinlan stopped the creature with a crushing punch to the throat. Gus advanced to the curb, hollering, "Get back, *cabrones*!" then aiming and letting the flaming bolt go, watching it drive through the smashed window frame and across the shop, landing in the rear wall.

Gus was racing away when the building shattered in a single blast. The brick face collapsed, spilling into the street, the roof and its wooden underpinnings bursting apart like the top paper of a firecracker.

The shockwave knocked the unaware vampires to the street. The suck of oxygen brought an odd, post-detonation silence to the block, which was compounded by the ringing in their ears.

Gus got to his knees, then his feet. The corner building was no more, flattened as though by a giant foot. Dust billowed out, the surviving vamps starting to rise all around them. Only those few who had been beaned by flying bricks stayed dead. The others recovered quickly from the blast, and once again turned their hungry gaze on the Sapphires.

From the corner of his eye, Gus saw Quinlan running away to the opposite side of the street, leaping down a short stairwell leading to a basement apartment. Gus didn't understand his retreat until he looked back to the destruction he had caused.

The explosive punch to the immediate atmosphere had rolled up to the smoke cover, the burst of moving air creating a rupture. A breach parted the blackness, allowing bright, cleansing sunlight to come pouring down.

The smoke opened, the sun line riding out from the impact site, spreading in a bright yellow cone of irradiating power—the dumb vamps sensing the impending rays only too late.

Gus watched them dissipate around him with ghostly screams. Their bodies fell, reduced instantaneously to steam and cinder. Those few who were at a safe distance from the sun turned and ran into neighboring buildings for cover.

Only the feelers reacted intelligently, anticipating the spreading sun and grabbing Bolivar. The little ones fought him, working together to drag him back from the approaching line of killing sun—just in time, yanking up a sidewalk vent grate and pulling him, clawing, down into the underground.

Suddenly the Sapphires and Angel and Gus were alone on a sunny street. They still had their weapons in hand, but no enemy stood before them.

Just another sunny day in East Harlem.

Gus went to the disaster area, the pawnshop blown off its foundation. The basement was now exposed, full of smoking bricks and settling dust. He called over Angel, who hobbled in to help Gus shift some of the heavier chunks of mortar, clearing a path. Gus climbed down into the wreckage, and Angel followed. He heard a sizzling sound, but it was just severed electrical connections still live with juice. He tossed aside a few chunks of brick, searching the floor for bodies, still concerned that the old man might have been hiding there the whole time.

No corpses. He didn't discover much of anything, really, just a lot of empty shelves. Almost as though the old man had recently cleared out. The door to the basement had been framed by the ultraviolet lamps now spitting orange sparks. Perhaps this had been a bunker of some sort, like a fallout shelter for a vampire attack—or else a kind of vault built to keep their kind out.

Gus lingered there longer than he should have—with the smoke seam already repairing itself, closing up on the sun once again—digging through the rubble for something, anything that might help him in his cause.

Concealed beneath a fallen wooden beam, Angel discovered, on its side, a small, sealed keepsake box made entirely of silver. A beautiful find. He lifted it up, showing it to the gang, and Gus in particular.

Gus took the box from him. "The old man," he said. And smiled.

Pennsylvania Station

WHEN THE OLD Pennsylvania Station opened in 1910, it had been considered a monument to excess. An opulent temple of mass transportation, and the largest interior space in all of New York, a city inclined toward excess even a century ago.

The demolition of the original station, which began in 1963, and its replacement by the current warren of tunnels and corridors, is viewed historically as a catalyst for the modern historical preservation movement, in that it was perhaps the first—and some say still the greatest—failure of "urban renewal."

Penn Station remained the busiest transportation hub in the United States, serving 600,000 passengers per day, four times as many as Grand Central Station. It served Amtrak, the Metropolitan Transportation Authority (MTA), and New

Jersey Transit—with a Port Authority Trans-Hudson (PATH) station just one block away, accessible back then by an underground passageway that had been now closed for many years for security reasons.

The modern Penn Station used the same underground platforms as the original Penn Station. Eph had booked Zack, Nora, and Nora's mother on the Keystone Service, straight through Philadelphia to its terminus, the state capital, Harrisburg. It was normally a four-hour trip, though significant delays were expected. Once there, Nora would survey the situation and arrange transportation to the girls' camp.

Eph left the van at an empty cab stand a block away and walked them through the quiet streets to the station. A dark cloud hung over the city, both literally and figuratively, smoke hovering ominously as they passed empty storefronts. Display windows were broken, and yet even the looters were gone—most of them turned into looters of human blood.

How far and how fast the city had fallen.

Only once they reached the Seventh Avenue entrance at Joe Louis Plaza, underneath the Madison Square Garden sign, did Eph recognize a hint of the New York of a few weeks ago, of last month. Cops and Port Authority workers in orange vests directed the downtrodden crowd, maintaining order as they moved them inside.

The stopped escalators allowed people down onto the concourse. The unceasing foot traffic had allowed the station to remain one of the last bastions of humanity in a city of vampires—resisting colonization despite its proximity to the underground. Eph was certain that most, if not all, trains were delayed, but it was enough that they were still running. The rush of panicked people reassured him. If the trains were stopped, this would have turned into a riot.

Few of the overhead lights were working. None of the stores were open, their shelves all empty, handwritten CLOSED UNTIL FURTHER NOTICE signs taped to the windows.

The groan of a train arriving on a lower platform reassured Eph as he shouldered Nora and Mrs. Martinez's bag, Nora seeing to it that her mother did not fall. The concourse was jammed, and yet he welcomed the press of the crowd; he had missed the feeling of being an organism surrounded by a throng of humanity.

National Guard soldiers waited up ahead, looking drawn and exhausted. Still, they were scanning faces as they went past, and Eph remained a wanted man.

Add to that the fact that he had Setrakian's silver-loaded pistol stuffed into the back of his waistband, and Eph accompanied them only as far as the great blue pillars, pointing out the Amtrak lounge gate around the bend.

Mariela Martinez looked scared and even somewhat angry. The crowd annoyed her. Nora's mother, a former home healthcare worker, had been diagnosed two years ago with early-onset Alzheimer's. Sometimes she thought Nora was sixteen years old, which occasionally led to trouble over who was in charge of whom. Today, however, she was quiet, overwhelmed and operating deep within herself, out of her element here and anxious about being away from home. No cross words for her departed husband; no insisting on getting dressed for a party. She wore a long raincoat over a saffron-colored housecoat, her hair hanging heavily behind her in a thick, gray braid. She had taken to Zack already, holding his hand on the ride in, which pleased Eph even as it tugged at his heart.

Eph knelt down in front of his son. The boy looked away, like he didn't want to do this, didn't want to say good-bye. "You help Nora with Mrs. Martinez, okay?"

Zack nodded. "Why does it have to be a girls' camp?"

"Because Nora is a girl and she went there. It's only going to be you three."

"And you," Zack said quickly. "When are you coming?"

"Very soon, I hope."

Eph had his hands on Zack's shoulders. Zack brought his hands up to grip Eph's forearms. "You promise?"

"Soon as I can."

"That's not a promise."

Eph squeezed his boy's shoulders, selling the lie. "I promise."

Zack wasn't buying it, Eph could tell. He could feel Nora looking down at them.

Eph said, "Gimme a hug."

"Why?" said Zack, pulling back a bit. "I'll hug you when I see you in Pennsylvania."

Eph flashed a smile. "One to tide me over then."

"I don't see why—"

Eph pulled him close, gripping him tightly while the crowd swirled past them. The boy struggled, but not really, and then Eph kissed his cheek and released him.

Eph stood and Nora pushed in front of him, gently backing Eph up two steps. Her brown eyes were fierce, right up in his. "Tell me now. What is this you are planning?"

"I'm going to say good-bye to you."

She stood close, like a lover saying farewell, only she had her knuckle pressed right into the lowest part of his sternum and was twisting it there like a screw. "After we're gone—what are you going to do? I want to know."

Eph looked past her at Zack, standing with Nora's mother, dutifully holding her hand. Eph said, "I'm going to try to stop this thing. What do you think?"

"I think it's too late for that, and you know it. Come with us. If you're doing this for the old man—I feel the same way about him you do. But it's over, we both know that. Come with us. We'll regroup there. We'll figure out our next move. Setrakian will understand."

Eph felt her pull on him more than the pain of her knuckle in his breastbone. "We still have a chance here," he said. "I believe that."

"We"—she made sure he saw that she was referring to the two of them—"still have a chance also, if we both get out of here now."

Eph pulled the last bag off his shoulder and hung it on hers. "Weapon bag," he said. "In case you run into any trouble."

Angry tears wet her eyes. "You should know that, if you end up doing something stupid here, I am determined to hate you forever."

He nodded once.

She kissed his lips, wrapping him in an embrace. Her hand found the butt of the pistol in the small of Eph's back, and her eyes darkened, her head moving back to study his face. For a moment Eph thought she was going to yank it out and take it from him, but instead she came close again, right up to his ear, her cheek wet with tears.

She whispered, "I hate you already."

She pulled away, not looking back at him as she gathered up Zack and her mother and ushered them toward the departures board.

Eph waited and watched Zack go, the boy looking back as they reached the corner, searching for him. Eph waved, his hand high—but the boy didn't see him. The Glock tucked inside Eph's belt suddenly felt heavier.

Inside the former headquarters of the Canary Project at Eleventh and 27th, the director of the Centers for Disease Control and Prevention, Dr. Everett Barnes, was napping in an office chair inside Ephraim Goodweather's old office. The ringing telephone penetrated his consciousness, but not enough to rouse him. It took the hand of an FBI special agent on his shoulder to do that.

Barnes sat up, shaking off sleep, feeling refreshed. "Washington?" he guessed.

The agent shook his head. "Goodweather."

Barnes pressed the flashing button on the desk phone and picked up the receiver. "Ephraim? Where are you?"

"Penn Station. Phone booth."

"Are you all right?"

"I just put my son on a train out of the city."

"Yes?"

"I'm ready to come in."

Barnes looked at the agent and nodded. "I am very relieved to hear that."

"I'd like to see you personally."

"Stay where you are, I am on my way."

He hung up and the agent handed him his coat. Barnes was attired in full Navy regalia. They went out the main office and down the steps to the curb, where Dr. Barnes's black SUV was parked. Barnes climbed into the passenger side and the agent started the ignition.

The blow came so suddenly, Barnes didn't know what was happening. Not to him—to the FBI agent. The man slumped forward, honking the horn with his chin. He tried to raise his hands and a second blow came—from the backseat. A hand wielding a pistol. It took one more blow to knock out the agent, leaving him slumped against the door.

The assailant was out of the backseat and opening the driver's door, pulling out the unconscious man and dumping him onto the sidewalk like a big bag of laundry.

Ephraim Goodweather leaped into the driver's seat and slammed the door. Barnes opened his door, but Eph pulled him back inside, jamming the gun against the inside of Barnes's thigh rather than his head. Only a doctor or perhaps a soldier knew that you might survive a head or neck wound, but one shot to the femoral artery meant certain death.

"Close it," said Eph.

Barnes did. Eph already had the SUV in drive, and was racing out onto 27th Street.

Barnes tried to squirm away from the pistol in his lap. "Please, Ephraim. Please let's talk—"

"Good! You start."

"May I at least put on my seat belt?"

Eph took the corner hard and said, "No."

Barnes saw that Ephraim had dumped something into the cup holders between them: the FBI agent's shield. The muzzle was tight against his leg, Eph's left hand heavy upon the steering wheel. "Please, Ephraim, be very, very careful—"

"Start talking, Everett." Eph pressed the gun hard into Barnes's leg. "Why the hell are you still here? Still in the city? You wanted a front-row seat, huh?"

"I don't know what you are referring to, Ephraim. This is where the sick are."

"The sick," said Eph disparagingly.

"The infected."

"Everett—you keep talking like that and this gun is going to go off."

"You've been drinking."

"And you've been lying. I want to know why there is *no goddamned quarantine*!" Eph's rage filled the interior of the car. He veered hard right to avoid a broken-down and looted delivery van. "No competent attempt at containment," he continued. "Why has this been allowed to keep burning? Answer me!"

Barnes was up against the door, whimpering like a boy. "It is completely out of my hands now!" he said.

"Let me guess. You are just following orders."

"I . . . I accept my role, Ephraim. The time came where a choice had to be made, and I made it. This world, the one we thought we knew, Ephraim—it is at the brink."

"You don't say."

Barnes's voice grew colder. "The smart bet is with them. Never wager with your heart, Ephraim. Every major institution has been compromised, either directly or indirectly. By that, I mean either corrupted or subverted. This is occurring at the highest levels."

Eph nodded hard. "Eldritch Palmer."

"Does it really matter at this point?"

"To me it does."

"When a patient is dying, Ephraim—when all hope for recovery is gone—what does a good physician do?"

"He keeps fighting."

"You prolong it? Really? When the end is certain and near? When they are already beyond saving—do you offer palliative care and draw out the inevitable? Or do you let nature run its course?"

"Nature! Jesus, Everett."

"I don't know what else to call it."

"I call it euthanasia. Of the entire human race. You standing back in your Navy uniform and watching it die on the table."

"You apparently want to make this personal, Ephraim, when I have caused none of this. Blame the disease, not the doctor. To a certain extent, I am as appalled as you are. But I am a realist, and some things simply cannot be wished away. I did what I did because there was no other choice."

"There is *always* a choice, Everett. Always. Fuck—I know that. But you . . . you are a coward, a traitor, and—worse—a fucking fool."

"You will lose this fight, Ephraim. In fact, if I'm not mistaken—you already have."

"We'll see about that," said Eph, already halfway across town. "You and I. We'll see it together."

Sotheby's

SOTHEBY'S, THE AUCTION house founded in 1744, brokered art, diamond, and international realty sales in forty countries, with principal salesrooms in London, Hong Kong, Paris, Moscow, and New York. Sotheby's New York occupied the length of York Avenue between 71st and 72nd Streets, one block in from FDR Drive and the East River. It was a glass-front, ten-story building, housing specialist departments, galleries, and auction spaces—some of which was normally open to the public.

Not this day, however. A private security detail wearing breathing masks were posted outside on the sidewalk and inside behind the revolving doors. The Upper East Side was attempting to maintain some semblance of civility, even as pockets of the city fell to chaos around them.

Setrakian expressed his desire to register as an approved bidder for the impending auction, and he and Fet were issued masks and allowed inside.

The building's front foyer was open, rising all the way to the top, ten levels of railed balconies going up. Setrakian and Fet were assigned an escort, and taken up escalators to a representative's office on the fifth floor.

The representative pulled on her paper mask as they entered, making no move to come out from behind her desk. Shaking hands was unsanitary. Setrakian reiterated his intention, and she nodded and produced a packet of forms.

"I need the name and number of your broker, and please list your securities accounts. Proof of intent to bid, in the form of an authorization for one million dollars, is the standard deposit for this level of auction."

Setrakian glanced at Fet, twiddling the pen in his crooked fingers. "I am afraid I am between brokers at present. I do, however, possess some interesting antiquities myself. I would be happy to put them up as collateral."

"I am very sorry." She was already retrieving the forms from him, refiling them in her desk drawers.

"If I might," said Setrakian, returning her pen, which she made no move to touch. "What I would really like to do is to view the catalog items before making a decision."

"I am afraid that is a privilege for bidders only. Security is very, very tight, as you probably know, due to some of the items being offered—"

"The *Occido Lumen*."

She swallowed. "Precisely, yes. There is much . . . much mystique surrounding the item, as you may be familiar with, and naturally, given the current state of affairs here in Manhattan . . . and the fact that no auction house has successfully offered the *Lumen* for sale in the past two centuries . . . well, one doesn't have to be especially superstitious to link the two."

"I am sure there is also a strong financial component. Why else go on with the auction at all? Evidently Sotheby's believes that its sale commission outweighs the risks associated with bringing the *Lumen* to auction."

"Well, I couldn't possibly comment on business affairs."

"Please." Setrakian laid a hand on the top edge of her desk, gently, as though it were her arm. "Is it at all possible? For an old man just to look?"

Her eyes were unmoved over her mask. "I cannot."

Setrakian looked to Fet. The city exterminator stood up and pulled down his mask. He produced his city badge. "Hate to do this, but—I need to see the building supervisor immediately. The person in charge of this property itself."

The director of Sotheby's North America rose from behind his desk when the building supervisor entered with Setrakian and Fet. "What is the meaning of this?"

The building supervisor said, his face mask puffing, "This gentleman says we have to evacuate the building."

"Evacuate the . . . what?"

"He has the authority to shutter the building for seventy-two hours while the city inspects it."

"Seventy-two . . . but what about the auction?"

"Canceled," said Fet. He punctuated that with a shrug. "Unless."

The director's expression flattened behind his mask, as though he suddenly understood. "This city is crumbling around us, and you choose now, today, to come looking for a bribe?"

"It's not a bribe I'm after," said Fet. "The truth is, and you can probably tell just by looking at me, I'm something of an art fanatic."

They were allowed restricted access to the *Occido Lumen*, their viewing occurring inside a private, glass-walled chamber within a larger viewing vault located behind two locked doors on the ninth floor. The bulletproof case was unlocked and removed, and Fet watched Setrakian prepare himself to inspect the long-sought tome, white cotton gloves covering his crooked hands.

The old book rested on an ornate viewing stand of white oak. It was 12 × 8 × 1.8 inches, 489 folios, handwritten in parchment, with twenty illuminated pages, bound in leather and faced with pure-silver plates on the front and rear covers and the spine. The pages themselves were also edged in silver.

Now it made sense to Fet. Why the book had never fallen into the possession of the Ancients. Why the Master didn't just come and take it from them right here, right now.

The silver casing. The book was literally beyond their grasp.

Twin cameras on arched stems rising out of the table captured images of the open pages, which were shown on oversized vertical plasma screens on the wall before them. The first illuminated page in the front matter featured a detailed drawing of a figure of six appendages done in fine, glowing silver leaf. The style and the minute calligraphy surrounding it spoke of another time, another world. Fet was drawn in by the reverence Setrakian showed this book. The quality of the craftsmanship impressed him, but, when it came to the artwork itself, Fet had no clue what he was looking at. He waited for insights from the old man. All he knew was that there were clear similarities between this work and the markings he and Eph had discovered in the subway. Even the three crescent moons were represented here.

Setrakian focused his interest on two pages,

one pure text, the other a rich illumination. Beyond the obvious artistry of the page, Fet could not understand what it was about the image that captivated the old man so—that wrung tears from Setrakian's eyes.

They stayed beyond their allotted fifteen minutes, Setrakian rushing to copy out some twenty-eight symbols. Only Fet could not find the symbols in the images on the page. But he said nothing, waiting while Setrakian—obviously frustrated by the stiffness of his crooked fingers—filled two sheets of paper with these symbols.

The old man was silent as they rode the elevator back down to the foyer. He said nothing until they had exited the building and were far enough away from the armed security guards.

Setrakian said, "The pages are watermarked. Only a trained eye can see it. Mine can."

"Watermarked? You mean, like currency?"

Setrakian nodded. "All the pages in the book. It was a common practice in some grimoires and alchemical treatises. Even in early tarot card sets. You see? There is text printed on the pages, but a second layer underneath. Watermarked directly into the paper at the time of its pressing. That is the real knowledge. The Sigil. The hidden symbol—the key . . ."

"Those symbols you copied . . ."

Setrakian patted his pocket, reassuring himself that he had taken the sketches with him.

He paused then, something catching his eye. Fet followed him across the street to the large building facing the glass front of Sotheby's. The

Mary Manning Walsh Home was a nursing home run by the Carmelite Sisters for the Archdiocese of New York.

Setrakian was drawn to the brick front to the left of the entrance awning. A graffiti design spray-painted there, in orange and black. It took Fet a moment to realize that it was yet another highly stylized, if cruder, variation on the illuminated figure in the front matter of the book locked away on the top floor of the facing building—a book no one had seen for decades.

"What the hell?" said Fet.

"It is him—his name," said Setrakian. "His true name. He is branding the city with it. Calling it his own."

Setrakian turned away, looking up at the black smoke blowing over the sky, obscuring the sun.

Setrakian said, "Now to find a way to get that book."

Extract from the diary of Ephraim Goodweather

Dearest Zack,

What you must know is that I needed to do this— not out of arrogance (I am no hero, son), but out of conviction. Leaving you in that train station—the pain I feel now is the worst I have ever experienced. Know that I never chose the human race instead of you. What I am to do now is for your future—yours alone. That the rest of mankind may benefit is but a side issue. This is so that you will never, ever have to do what I just did: choose between your child and your duty.

From the moment I first held you in my arms, I knew that you were going to be the only genuine love story in my life. The one human being to whom I could give my all and expect nothing in return. Please understand that I cannot trust anyone else to attempt what I am about to do. Much of the history of the previous century was written with a gun. Written by men driven to murder by their conviction, and their demons. I have both. Insanity is real, son—it is existence now. No longer a disorder of the mind, but an external reality. Maybe I can change this.

I will be branded a criminal, I may be called mad—but my hope is that, in time, the truth will vindicate my name, and that you, Zachary, will once again hold me in your heart.

No amount of words will ever do justice to what I feel for you and the relief that you are now safe with Nora. Please think of your father not as a man who deserted you, who broke a promise to you, but as a man who wanted to ensure that you survived this assault on our species. As a man with difficult choices to make, just like the man you will one day grow to be.

Please think also of your mother—as she was. Our love for you will never die so long as you live. In you, we have given this world a great gift—and of that, I have no doubt.

Your old man,
Dad

Office of Emergency Management, Brooklyn

THE OFFICE OF Emergency Management building operated on a darkened block in Brooklyn. The four-year-old, $50 million OEM facility served as the central point of coordination for major emergencies in New York. It housed New York's 130-agency Emergency Operations Center, containing state-of-the-art audiovisual and information technology systems and full backup generators. The headquarters had been built to replace the agency's former facility at 7 World Trade Center, destroyed on 9/11. It was constructed to foster resource coordination between public agencies in the event of a large-scale disaster. To that end, redundant electromechanical systems ensured continuous operation during a power outage.

The twenty-four-hours-a-day building was operating exactly as it should. The problem was that many of the agencies it was meant to coordinate with—local, state, federal, and nonprofit—were either offline, understaffed, or else apparently abandoned.

The heart of the city's emergency disaster network was still beating strong, but precious little of its informational blood was reaching the extremities—as if the city had suffered a massive stroke.

Eph feared he would miss his narrow window of opportunity. Getting back across the bridge took him much longer than he had expected: most people who were able and willing to leave Manhattan had already done so, and the road debris and abandoned cars made the crossing difficult. Someone had tied two corners of an immense yellow tarpaulin to one of the bridge's support wires, rippling in the wind like an old maritime flag of quarantine flying off the mast of a doomed ship.

Director Barnes sat quietly, gripping the handle over the window, finally realizing that Eph was not going to tell him where they were headed.

The Long Island Expressway was substantially faster, Eph eyeing the towns as he passed them, seeing empty streets from the overpasses, quiet gas stations, empty mall parking lots.

His plan was dangerous, he knew. More desperate than organized. A psychopath's plan, perhaps. But he was okay with this: insanity was all around him. And sometimes luck trumped preparation.

He arrived just in time to catch the beginning of Palmer's address on the car radio. He parked near a train station, turning off the engine, turning to Barnes.

"Get out your ID now. We're going inside the OEM together. I will have the gun under my jacket. You say anything to anybody or try to alert security, I will shoot whoever you talk to and then I will shoot you. Do you believe me?"

Barnes looked into Eph's eyes. He nodded.

"Now we walk, and fast."

They came up on the OEM building along 15th

Street, the road lined with official vehicles on both sides. The tan-brick building exterior resembled that of a new grade school, nearly a block long but only two stories tall. A broadcast tower rose behind it, surrounded by a wire-topped fence. National Guard members stood at ten-yard intervals along the short lawn, securing the building.

Eph saw the gated parking lot entrance, and, inside, what had to be Palmer's idling motorcade. The middle limousine appeared almost presidential, and certainly bulletproof.

He knew he must get Palmer before he got into that car.

"Walk tall," said Eph, his hand around Barnes's elbow, steering him along the sidewalk past the soldiers toward the entrance.

A group of protesters heckled them from across the street, holding signs about God's wrath, proclaiming that because America had lost faith in Him, He was now abandoning it. A preacher in a shabby suit stood atop a short stepladder, reading verses out of Revelation. Those surrounding him stood with their open palms facing the OEM in a gesture of blessing, praying over the city agency. One placard featured a hand-drawn icon of a downcast Jesus Christ bleeding from a crown of thorns, sporting vampire fangs and glaring red eyes.

"Who will deliver us now?" the shabby monk cried.

Sweat ran down Eph's chest, past the silver-loaded pistol stuck in his belt.

* * *

Eldritch Palmer sat in the Emergency Operations Center before a microphone set upon a table and a pitcher of water. He faced a video wall upon which was displayed the seal of the United States Congress.

Alone, except for his trusted aide, Mr. Fitzwilliam, Palmer wore his usual dark suit, looking a shade paler than usual, a bit more shrunken in the chair. His wrinkled hands rested on the top of the table, still, waiting.

Via satellite link, he was about to address an emergency joint session of the United States Congress. This unprecedented address, with questions to follow, was also being broadcast via live Internet feed over all television and radio networks and their affiliates still in operation, and internationally across the globe.

Mr. Fitzwilliam stood just out of camera view, his hands clasped at belt level, looking outside the secure room into the larger facility. Most of the 130 workstations were occupied, and yet no work was being done. All eyes were turned to the hanging monitors.

After brief opening remarks, facing the half-full Capitol chamber, Palmer read from a prepared statement scrolling in large print on a teleprompter behind the camera.

"I want to address this public health emergency in terms of where myself and my Stoneheart Group are well-positioned to intervene, to respond, to reassure. What I can present to you today is a three-fold action plan for the United States of America, and the world beyond.

"First, I am pledging an immediate loan of three billion dollars to the city of New York, in order to keep city services functioning and to fund a citywide quarantine.

"Second, as the president and CEO of Stoneheart Industries, I want to extend my personal guarantee as to the capacity and security of this nation's food delivery system, both through our essential transportation holdings and our various meatpacking facilities.

"Third, I would respectively recommend that the remaining Nuclear Regulatory Commission procedures be suspended in order that the completed Locust Valley Nuclear Power Plant be allowed to come online immediately, as a direct solution to New York's current catastrophic power-grid problems."

As head of the Canary Project in New York, Eph had been inside the OEM a few times before. He was familiar with the entrance procedures, which were secure and yet manned by armed professionals used to dealing with other armed professionals. So while Barnes's identification was inspected rather closely, Eph simply dropped his shield and pistol into a basket and walked briskly through the metal detector.

"Would you like an escort, Director Barnes?" asked the security guard.

Eph grabbed his things and Barnes's arm. "We know the way."

Palmer's questioning fell to a panel of three Democrats and two Republicans. He faced the most scrutiny from the ranking member of the Department of Homeland Security, Representative Nicholas Frone of the Third Congressional District of New York, also a member of the House Financial Committee. Voters were said not to trust baldness or beards, and yet, on both counts, Frone had bucked the trend now for three successive terms of office.

"As to this quarantine, Mr. Palmer—I have to say, hasn't that horse already left the barn?"

Palmer sat with his hands set upon a single piece of paper in front of him. "I enjoy your folksy sayings, Representative Frone. But as someone who grew up in the seat of privilege, you might not realize that it is indeed possible for an industrious farmer to saddle and mount another horse in order to safely rein in the one that got away. America's working farmers would never give up on a good horse. I think neither should we."

"Also I find it interesting that you should tie your pet project, this nuclear reactor, that you have been trying to ram through regulatory procedures, into your proposal. I'm not at all convinced this is a good time to be rushing such a plant into production. And I would like to know how exactly it will help, when the problem, as I understand it, is not energy deficiency but interruptions in delivery."

Palmer responded, "Representative Frone, two critical power plants servicing New York State are currently offline, due to voltage overload and power-line failure caused by widespread surges in the system. This starts a chain reaction of adverse effects. It decreases the water supply, due to a lack of pressure in the lines, which will lead to contamination if it is not immediately addressed. It has impacted rail transportation up and down the northeast corridor, the safe screening of passengers for air transportation, and even road travel, with the unavailability of electric gasoline pumps. It has disrupted mobile telephone communication, which impacts statewide emergency services, such as 911 response, placing citizens directly at risk."

Palmer continued, "Now, as to nuclear power, this plant, located in your district, is ready to come online. It has passed every preliminary regulation without flaw, and yet bureaucratic procedures demand more waiting. You have a fully capable power plant—one that you yourself campaigned against and resisted every step of the way—that could power much of the city if activated. A hundred and four such plants supply twenty percent of this country's electricity, and yet this is the first nuclear power plant to have been commissioned in the United States since the Three Mile Island incident in 1978. The word 'nuclear' dredges up negative connotations, but, in fact, it is a sustainable energy source that reduces carbon emissions. It is our only honest large-scale alternative to fossil fuels."

Representative Frone said, "Let me interrupt your commercial message here, Mr. Palmer. With all due respect, isn't this crisis nothing more than a fire sale for the superrich such as yourself? Pure 'Shock Doctrine,' is it not? I, for one, am very curious to know what you plan to do with New York City once you own it."

"As I made clear previously, this would be an interest-free, twenty-year revolving line of credit . . ."

Eph dumped the FBI credentials in a wastebasket and continued with Barnes through the Emergency Operations Center that was the heart of the facility. The attention of everyone present was focused on Palmer, pictured on the many monitors overhead.

Eph saw dark-suited Stoneheart men clustered around a side hall leading to a pair of glass doors. The sign with the arrow read: SECURE CONFERENCE ROOM.

A chill washed over Eph, as he realized he was almost certain to die here. Certainly if he succeeded. Indeed, his worst fear was that he might be cut down without successfully assassinating Eldritch Palmer.

Eph guessed the direction of the parking lot exit. He turned to Barnes and whispered, "Act sick."

"What?"

"Act sick. Shouldn't be too much of a stretch for you."

Eph continued with him past the conference-room hall toward the rear. Another Stoneheart man stood near a pair of doors. Before him hung a glowing sign for the men's restroom.

"Here it is, sir," said Eph, opening the door for Barnes. Barnes entered holding his belly, clearing his throat into his wrist. Eph rolled his eyes at the Stoneheart, whose facial expression did not change at all.

Inside the restroom, they were alone. Palmer's words carried over speakers. Eph pulled out the gun. He walked Barnes into the farthest stall and sat him on the covered toilet.

"Get comfortable," he said.

"Ephraim," said Barnes. "They are certain to kill you."

"I know," Eph said, pistol-whipping Barnes before closing the door. "That's what I came here for."

Representative Frone continued, "Now, there were reports in the media, before all this began, that you and your minions had been undertaking a raid on the world silver market, trying to corner it. Frankly, there have been many wild stories regarding this outbreak. Some of them—true or not—have struck a chord. Plenty of people believe it. Are you, in fact, preying on people's fears and superstitions? Or is this, as I hope, the lesser of two evils—a simple case of greed?"

Palmer picked up the piece of paper before him. He folded it once lengthwise, then once again across, and carefully slid the page into his inside breast pocket. He did so slowly, his eyes never leaving the camera connecting him to Washington, DC.

"Representative Frone, I believe that this is exactly the kind of pettiness and moral gridlock that has led us to this dark time. It is a matter of record that I have donated the maximum amount allowable by law to your opponent in each of your previous campaigns, and this is how you take—"

Frone yelled over him, "That's an outrageous charge!"

"Gentlemen," said Palmer, "you see before you an old man. A frail man, with very little time left on this earth. A man who wants to give back to the nation that has given him so very much in his life. Now I find myself in a unique position to do just that. Within the boundaries of the law— never above it. No one is above the law. Which is why I wanted to make a full accounting before you today. Please allow a patriot's final act to be a noble one. That is all. Thank you."

Mr. Fitzwilliam pulled out his chair, and Palmer got to his feet amid the hubbub and gavel-banging from the chamber on the video wall before him.

Eph stood by the door, listening. Movement outside, but not enough hubbub yet. He was tempted to open the door just a bit, but it opened inward, and he would certainly have been seen.

He tugged on the pistol's handle, keeping it loose and ready in his waistband.

A man walked past, saying, as though into a radio, "Get the car."

That was Eph's cue. He took a deep breath and reached for the door handle, walking out of the restroom and into murder.

Two Stonehearts in dark suits were moving to the far end of the hall, the doors leading outside. Eph turned the other way, seeing two more rounding the corner, advance men, eyeing him immediately.

Eph's timing had been less than perfect. He stepped to the side, as though deferring to the men, trying to appear uninterested.

Eph saw the small front wheels first. A wheelchair was being rolled around the corner. Two polished shoes were set on the fold-down footrests.

It was Eldritch Palmer, looking exceedingly small and frail. His flour-white hands were folded in his sunken lap, his eyes looking straight ahead, not at Eph.

One of the advance men veered off toward Eph, as though to block his view of the passing billionaire. Palmer was fewer than five yards away. Eph could not wait any longer.

His heart racing, Eph pulled the gun from his waistband. Everything happened in slow motion and all at once.

Eph raised the gun and darted to the left, in order to clear the Stoneheart man in his way. His hand trembled, but his arm was straight, his aim true.

He aimed for the largest target—the chest of the seated man—and squeezed the trigger. But the lead Stoneheart man threw himself at Eph—sacrificing himself more automatically than any Secret Service agent had ever leaped in front of a U.S. president.

The round struck the man in the chest, thudding off the body armor beneath his suit. Eph reacted just in time, shoving the man to the side before he could be tackled.

Eph fired again, but off-balance, the silver bullet ricocheting off Palmer's wheelchair armrest.

Eph fired again, but the Stonehearts threw themselves in front of Palmer. The third round went into the wall. An especially large man with a military crew cut—the man pushing Palmer's chair—started to run, wheeling his benefactor forward so that the Stoneheart men were catapulted onto Eph, and he went down.

He twisted as he fell, his gun arm facing the exit doorway. One more shot. He raised it to fire at the back of the chair, around the large bodyguard—but a shoe stomped down on his forearm, the round firing into the carpet, the weapon leaping from Eph's grip.

Eph was at the bottom of a growing pile, bodies rushing in from the main room now. Shouts, screams. Hands clawing at Eph, pulling at his limbs. He twisted his head just enough to see, through the arms and legs of his attackers, the wheelchair being pushed out through the double doors, into blazing daylight.

Eph howled in agony. His only chance gone forever. The moment slipping away.

The old man had survived unharmed.

Now the world was nearly his.

The Black Forest Solutions Facility

THE MASTER, STANDING at full height inside the utter blackness of a large chamber deep beneath the meatpacking plant, was electrically alert with meditative focus. It had become more deliberative as its sun-scorched flesh continued to flake off its once-human host body, exposing raw, red dermis beneath.

The Master's head rotated a few degrees on its great, broad neck, turning slightly toward the entrance, giving Bolivar its attention. No need for Bolivar to report what the Master already knew, what the Master had already—through Bolivar—seen: the arrival of the human hunters at the pawnshop, evidently in hopes of contacting old Setrakian, and the disastrous battle that ensued.

Behind Bolivar, feelers skittered about on all four limbs, like blind crabs. They "saw" something that unsettled them, as Bolivar was learning to infer from their behavior.

Someone was coming. The feelers' disquiet was offset by the Master's distinct lack of concern about the interloper.

The Master said: *The Ancient Ones have employed mercenaries for day hunting. A further sign of their desperation. And the old professor?*

Bolivar said: *He slipped away in advance of our attack. Inside his domicile, the feelers sensed that he is still alive.*

Hiding. Plotting. Scheming.

With the same desperation as the Ancients.

Humans only become dangerous when they have nothing to lose.

The whir of a motorized wheelchair, and the sound of its nubby tires rolling over the dirt floor, announced that the visitor was Eldritch Palmer. His bodyguard nurse trailed him, holding blue glow sticks to illuminate the passage for their human vision.

Feelers skittered away at the wheelchair's advance, crawling halfway up the wall, remaining outside the glow radius of the chemical luminescence, hissing.

"More creatures," said Palmer under his breath, unable to hide his distaste upon seeing the blind vampire children and their black-eyed stares. The billionaire was furious. "Why this hole?"

It pleases me.

Palmer saw, for the first time, by the light of the soft blue glow, the Master's flesh peeling. Chunks of it littered the ground at his feet like shorn hair beneath a barber's chair. Palmer was troubled by the sight of the raw flesh revealed beneath the Master's cracked exterior, and got to talking quickly, in order that the Master not read his mind like a soothsayer divining through a crystal ball.

"Look here. I have waited and I have done everything you've asked and I have received nothing in return. Now an attempt has been made on my life! I want my reward now! My patience has reached its end. You will give me what I am promised, or I will bankroll you no longer—do you understand? This is the end of it!"

The Master's skin crinkled as its ceiling-scraping head leaned forward. The monster was indeed intimidating, but Palmer would not back down.

"My premature death, should it come, would render this entire plan moot. You will have no more leverage upon my will—nor claim upon my resources."

Eichhorst, the perverse Nazi commandant, summoned to the chamber by the Master, entered behind Palmer into the haze of blue light. *You would do well to hold your human tongue in the presence of* Der Meister.

The Master, with a wave of his great hand, silenced Eichhorst. His red eyes appeared purple in the blue light, fixing wide on Palmer. *So it is done. I will grant your wish for immortality. In one day's time.*

Palmer stammered, taken aback. First, because of his surprise at the Master's sudden capitulation—after all these years of effort. And then, in recognition of the great leap Palmer was poised to take. To dive into the abyss that is death, and surface on the other side . . .

The businessman inside of him wanted more of a guarantee. But the schemer inside of him held his tongue.

You do not place provisions on a monster such

as the Master. You bid for its favor, and then accept its largesse with gratitude.

One more mortal day. Palmer thought he might even enjoy it.

All plans are fully in motion. My Brood is marching across the mainland. We have exposure in every critical destination, our circle widening in cities and provinces around the globe.

Palmer swallowed his anticipation, saying, "And even as the circle grows, it simultaneously tightens." His old hands described the scenario, fingers interlocking, palms squeezing together in a pantomime of strangling.

Indeed. One last task that remains before the start of The Devouring.

Eichhorst, looking like half a man beside the giant Master, said: *The book.*

"Of course," said Palmer. "It will be yours. But, I must ask you . . . if you already know the contents . . ."

It is not critical that I be in possession of the book. It is critical that others are not.

"So—why not just blow up the auction house? Explode the entire block?"

Crude solutions have been attempted in the past, and have failed. This book has had too many lives. I must be absolutely certain of its fate. So that I may watch it burn.

The Master then straightened to its full height, becoming distracted in such a way that only the Master could.

It was seeing something. The Master was physically in the cave with them, but psychically it was seeing through another's eyes—one of the Brood.

Into Palmer's head, the Master uttered two words:

The boy.

Palmer waited for an explanation, which never came. The Master had returned to the present, the now. He had returned to them with a new certainty, as if he had glimpsed the future.

Tomorrow the world burns and the boy and the book will be mine.

Fet's Blog

I HAVE KILLED.

I have slain.

With the hands typing this now.

I have stabbed, sliced, beat, crushed, dismembered, beheaded.

I have worn their white blood on my clothes and my boots.

I have destroyed. And I have rejoiced at the destruction.

You may say, as an exterminator by trade, I've been training for this all my life.

I understand the argument. I just can't support it.

Because it is one thing to have a rat race up your arm in blind fear.

Yet quite another to face a fellow human form and cut it down.

They look like people. They are very much like you and me.

I am no longer an exterminator. I am a vampire hunter.

And here is the other thing.

Something I will only say here, because I don't dare tell anyone else.

Because I know what they will think.

I know what they will feel.

I know what they will see when they look into my eyes.

But—all this killing?

I kind of like it.

And I'm good at it.

I might even be great at it.

The city is falling and probably the world. Apocalypse is a big word, a heavy word, when you realize you are actually facing it.

I can't be the only one. There must be others out there like me. People who have lived their whole lives feeling half-complete. Who never truly fit anywhere in the world. Who never understood why they were here, or what they were meant for. Who never answered the call, because they never heard it. Because nothing ever spoke to them.

Until now.

Penn Station

NORA LOOKED AWAY for what seemed like only a moment. As she stared at the big board, waiting for their track number to be announced, her gaze deepened and, utterly exhausted, she zoned out.

For the first time in days, she thought of nothing. No vampires, no fears, no plans. She relaxed her focus, and her mind dipped into sleep mode while her eyes remained open.

When she blinked back to awareness, it was like waking up from a dream about falling. A shudder, a startle. A small gasp.

She turned and saw Zack next to her, listening to his iPod.

But her mother was gone.

Nora looked around, didn't see her. She tugged down Zack's earbuds, asking him, and he joined her in looking.

"Wait here," said Nora, pointing to their bags. "Do not move!"

She pushed her way through the shoulder-to-shoulder crowd waiting before the departures board. She looked for a seam in the crowd, some path her slow-moving mother might have left, but saw nothing.

"Mama!"

Raised voices made Nora turn. She pushed toward them, coming out of the dense crowd near the side of the concourse, by the gate of a closed deli.

There was her mother, haranguing a bewildered-looking family of South Asians.

"Esme!" yelled Nora's mother, invoking the name of her late sister, Nora's late aunt. "Take care of the kettle, Esme! It's boiling, I can hear it!"

Nora reached her finally, taking her arm, stammering an apology to the non-English-speaking parents and their two young daughters. "Mama, come."

"There you are, Esme," she said. "What's that burning?"

"Come, Mama." Tears wet Nora's eyes.

"You're burning down my house!"

Nora clasped her mother's arm and pulled her back through the crowd, ignoring the grunts and insults. Zack was on tiptoes, looking for them. Nora said nothing to him, not wanting to break down in front of the boy. But this was too much. Everybody has a breaking point. Nora was fast approaching hers.

How proud her mother had been of her daughter, first a chemistry major at Fordham, then medical school with a specialty in bio-chem at Johns Hopkins. Nora saw now that her mother must have assumed she had it made. A rich doctor for a daughter. But Nora's interest had been public health, not internal medicine or pediatrics. Looking back now, she thought that growing up in the shadow of Three Mile Island had shaped her life more than she had realized. The Centers for Disease Control and Prevention paid government grade, a far cry from the healthy income potential of many of her peers. But she was young—there was time to serve now and earn later.

Then her mother got lost one day on the way to the grocery store. Having trouble tying her shoes, turning on the oven and walking away. Now conversing with the dead. The Alzheimer's diagnosis prompted Nora to give up her own apartment, in order to care for her declining mother. She had been putting off finding a suitable long-term-care facility for her, mainly because she still did not know how she could afford it.

Zack noticed Nora's distress but left her alone, sensing that she did not want to discuss it. He disappeared back beneath his earbuds.

Then suddenly, hours after it was scheduled, the track number for their train finally flipped over on the big board, announcing the train's approach. A mad rush ensued. Shoving and yelling, stiff-arming, name-calling. Nora gathered up their bags and hooked her mother's arm and hollered at Zack to move.

It got uglier still when the Amtrak official at the top of the narrow escalator leading down to the track said the train wasn't ready yet. Nora found herself near the rear of the angry crowd—so far back, she wasn't sure they would make it onto the train, even with paid tickets.

And so, Nora did something she had promised herself she would never do: she used her CDC badge to push her way through to the front of the line. She did so knowing that it was not for her own selfish benefit but for her mother and Zack. Still, she heard the name-calling and felt the daggers in every passenger's eyes as the crowd slowly parted, begrudgingly allowing them through.

And then it seemed it was all for nothing. Once they finally opened the escalator and allowed passengers down to the underground track, Nora found herself facing empty rails. The train was again delayed, and no one would tell them why, or give an estimate as to how long.

Nora arranged for her mother to sit on their

bags at their prime position at the yellow line. She and Zack split the last of a bag of Hostess doughnuts, Nora allowing each of them only sips of water from the half-full gym bottle she had packed.

The afternoon had slipped away from them. They would be departing—fingers crossed—after sunset, and that made Nora nervous. She had planned and expected to be well out of the city and on their way west by nightfall. She kept leaning out over the edge of the platform, eyeing the tunnels, her weapon bag tight against her side.

The rush of tunnel air came like a sigh of relief. The light announced the train's approach, and everyone stood. Nora's mother was nearly elbowed over the edge by some guy wearing an enormously bulky backpack. The train glided in, everyone jockeying for position—as a pair of doors miraculously stopped right in front of Nora. Finally something was going their way.

The doors parted and the rush of the crowd carried them inside. She claimed twin seats for her mother and Zack, shoving their possessions into the overhead rack, save for Zack's backpack—he held it on his lap—and Nora's weapon bag. Nora stood before them, their knees touching hers, hands gripping the railing overhead.

The rest piled inside. Once aboard, and knowing now that the final stage of their exodus was about to begin, the relieved passengers exhibited a bit more civility. Nora watched a man give up his seat to a woman with a child. Strangers helped others hauling bags. There was an immediate sense of community among the fortunate.

Nora herself felt a sudden sense of well-being. She was at least on the verge of breathing easy. "You good?" she asked Zack.

"Never better," he said, with a slight roll of his eyes, untangling his iPod wires and fitting the buds into his ears.

As she had feared, many passengers—some of them ticketed, some unticketed—did not make the train. After some trouble closing all the doors, those left behind began banging on the windows, while others went pleading to attendants who looked like they would rather be on the train themselves. Those that had been turned away looked like war-torn refugees, and Nora closed her eyes and said a brief prayer for them—and then another one for herself, for forgiveness, for putting her loved ones ahead of these strangers.

The silver train started to move west, toward the tunnels under the Hudson River, and the packed car broke out into applause. Nora watched the lights of the station slide away and disappear, and then they were rising through the underworld, toward the surface—like swimmers surfacing for much-needed breath.

She felt good inside the train, cutting through the darkness like a sword through a vampire. She looked down at her mother's lined face, watching the woman's eyes dip and flutter. Two minutes of rocking put her immediately to sleep.

They emerged from the station into the fallen night, running briefly aboveground before the tunnels underneath the Hudson River. As rain spit at the train's windows, Nora gasped at what she saw. Glimpses of anarchy: cars in flames, distant blazes, people fighting under strings of black rain. People running through the streets—were they being chased? Hunted? Were they even people at all? Maybe they were the ones doing the hunting.

She checked Zack, finding him focused on his iPod display. Nora saw, in his concentration, the father in the son. Nora loved Eph, and believed she could love Zack—even though she still knew so little about him. Eph and his boy were similar in so many ways, beyond appearance. She and Zack would have plenty of time to get to know each other once they reached the isolated camp.

She looked back out at the night, the darkness, and the power outages broken here and there by headlights, occasional bursts of generator-powered illumination. Light equaled hope. The land on either side began to give way, the city starting to retreat. Nora pressed against the window to chart their progress, to gauge how long it would be until they were through the next tunnel and clear of New York.

That was when she saw, standing on the top corner of a low wall, a figure outlined against a spray of upturned light. Something about this apparition made Nora quiver, a premonition of evil. She could not take her eyes off the figure as the train approached . . . and the figure began to raise its arm.

It was pointing at the train. Not just at the train, it seemed—but directly at Nora.

The train slowed as it passed, or maybe that was only how it seemed to Nora, her sense of time and motion bent by terror.

Smiling, backlit in the rain, hair sleek and dirty, mouth horribly distended and red eyes ablaze—Kelly Goodweather stared at Nora Martinez.

Their eyes locked as the train rolled past. Kelly's finger followed Nora.

Nora pressed her forehead against the glass, sickened by the sight of the vampire, and yet knowing what Kelly was about to do.

Kelly jumped at the last moment, leaping with preternatural animal grace, disappearing from Nora's sight as she latched on to the train.

The Flatlands

SETRAKIAN WORKED QUICKLY, hearing Fet's van arrive at the back of the shop. He flipped madly through the pages of the old volume on the table, this one the third volume of the French edition of *Collection des anciens alchimistes grecs*, published by Berthelot and Ruelle in Paris in 1888, his eyes going back and forth between its engraved pages and the sheets of symbols he had copied from the *Lumen*. He studied one symbol in particular. He finally located the engraving, his hands and eyes stopping for a moment.

A six-winged angel, wearing a crown of thorns, with a face both blind and mouthless—but with multiple mouths festooning each of its wings. At its feet was a familiar symbol—a crescent moon—and a single word.

"Argentum," read Setrakian. He gripped the yellowing page reverently—and then tore the engraving from its old binding, jamming it inside the pages of his notebook, just as Fet opened the door.

F et was back before sundown. He was certain he had not been found or traced by the vampire brood, which would lead the Master straight back to Setrakian.

The old man was working over a table near the radio, closing up one of his old books. He had tuned in a talk show, playing low, one of the few voices still on the airwaves. Fet felt a true affinity for Setrakian. Part of it was the bond that grows between soldiers in times of battle, the brotherhood of the trench—in this case, the trench being New York City. Then there was the great respect Fet felt for this weakened old man who simply would not stop fighting. Fet liked to think there were similarities between himself and the professor, in their dedication to a vocation, and mastery of knowledge about their foes—the obvious difference being one of scope, in that Fet fought pests and nuisance animals, while Setrakian had committed himself, at a young age, to eradicating an inhuman race of parasitic beings.

In one sense, Fet thought of himself and Eph as the professor's surrogate sons. Brothers in arms, yet as opposite as could be. One was a healer, the other an exterminator. One a university-trained family man of high status, the other a blue-collar, self-educated loner. One lived in Manhattan, the other Brooklyn.

And yet the one who had originally been at the forefront of the outbreak, the medical scientist, had seen his influence fall away in the dark days since the source of the virus had become known. While his opposite number, the city employee with a little sideline shop in Flatlands—and the killer instinct—now served at the old man's side.

There was one other reason Fet felt close to Setrakian. Something Fet could not bring up to him, nor something he was entirely clear on himself. Fet's parents had immigrated to this country from the Ukraine (not Russia, as they told people, and as Fet still claimed), not only in search of the opportunities all immigrants seek but also to escape their past. Fet's father's father—and this was nothing he had ever been told, because no one in his family spoke of it directly, especially his sour father—had been a Soviet prisoner of war, who was conscripted into service at one of the extermination camps during World War II. Whether it was Treblinka or Sobibor or elsewhere, Fet did not know. It was nothing he ever desired to explore. His grandfather's role in the Shoah was revealed two decades after the war ended, and he was jailed. In his defense, he claimed that he had been victimized at the hands of the Nazis, forced into the lowly role of camp guard. Ukrainians of German extraction had been installed in positions of authority, while the rest toiled at the whim of the sadistic camp commanders. Yet prosecutors submitted evidence of personal enrichment in the postwar years, such as the source of Fet's grandfather's wealth in starting his dressmaking company, which he was unable to explain. But it was a blurred photograph of him wearing a black uniform, standing against a fence of barbed wire with a carbine in his gloved hands—lips curled in an expression claimed by some to be a nasty smirk, by others a grimace—that ultimately did him in. Fet's father never spoke of it while he was alive. What little Fet knew, he had learned from his mother.

Shame can indeed be visited upon future generations, and Fet carried this with him now like a terrible burden, a hot dose of shame always in the pit of his stomach. Realistically, a man can bear no responsibility for the actions of his grandfather, and yet . . .

And yet one carries the sins of his forebears as one carries their features in his face. One bears their blood, and their honor or their blight.

Fet had never suffered from this affiliation as he did now—except perhaps in dreams. One sequence recurred, disrupting his sleep again and again. In it, Fet has returned to his family's home village, a place he had never visited in real life. Every door and window is shut to him, and he walks the streets alone, yet watched. And then suddenly, from one end of the street, a roaring burst of angry orange light flies toward him on the cadence of galloping hooves.

A stallion—its coat, mane, and tail aflame—is

charging at him. The horse is fully consumed, and Fet, always at the very last second, dives out of its path, turning and watching the animal tear off across the countryside, trailing dark smoke in its wake.

"How is it out there?"

Fet set down his satchel. "Quiet. Menacing." He shrugged off his jacket, pulling a jar of peanut butter and some Ritz crackers from the pockets. He had stopped off at his apartment. He offered some to Setrakian. "Any word?"

"Nothing," said Setrakian, inspecting the cracker box as though he might turn down the snack. "But Ephraim is long overdue."

"The bridges. Clogged."

"Mmm." Setrakian pulled out the wax wrapper, sniffing at the contents before trying a cracker. "Did you get the maps?"

Fet patted his pocket. He had journeyed to a DPW depot in Gravesend in order to procure sewer maps for Manhattan, specifically the Upper East Side. "I got them, all right. Question is—will we get to use them?"

"We will. I am certain."

Fet smiled. The old man's faith never failed to warm him. "Can you tell me what you saw in that book?"

Setrakian set down the box of crackers and lit up a pipe. "I saw . . . everything. I saw hope, yes. But then . . . I saw the end of us. Of everything."

He slid out a reproduction of the crescent moon drawing seen both in the subway, via Fet's pink phone video, and in the pages of the *Lumen*. The old man had copied it three times.

"You see? This symbol—like the vampire itself, how it was once seen—is an archetype. Common to all mankind, East and West—but within it, a different permutation, see? Latent, but revealed in time, like any prophecy. Observe."

He took the three pieces of paper and, utilizing a makeshift light table, laid them out, superimposing one atop another.

"Any legend, any creature, any symbol we ever stumble on, already exists in a vast cosmic reservoir where archetypes wait. Shapes looming outside our Platonic cave. We naturally believe ourselves clever and wise, so advanced, and those who came before us so naïve and simple . . . when all we truly do is echo the order of the universe, as it guides us . . ."

The three moons rotated in the paper, and joined together.

"These are not three moons. No. They are occultations. Three solar eclipses, each occurring at the exact latitude and longitude, marking an even, enormous span of years—signaling an event, now complete. Revealing the sacred geometry of omen."

Fet saw with amazement that the three shapes together formed a rudimentary biohazard sign: ☣. "But this symbol . . . I know it from my work. It was just designed in the sixties, I think . . ."

"All symbols are eternal. They exist even before we dream of them . . ."

"So how did . . ."

"Oh, we know," said Setrakian. "We always know. We don't discover, we don't learn. We just remember things that we have forgotten . . ." He pointed to the symbol. "A warning. Dormant in our mind, reawakened now—as the end of time approaches."

Fet regarded the worktable Setrakian had taken over. He was experimenting with photography equipment, explaining something about "testing a metallurgical silver emulsion technique" that Fet did not understand. But the old man seemed to know what he was doing. "Silver," said Setrakian. "*Argentum,* to the ancient alchemists and represented by this symbol . . ." Again, Setrakian presented Fet with the image of the crescent moon.

"And this, in turn . . ." said Setrakian, producing the engraving of the archangel. "Sariel. In certain Enochian manuscripts he is named Arazyal, Asaradel. Names all too similar to Azrael or Ozryel . . ."

Placing the engraving side to side with the biohazard sign and the alchemical symbol of the crescent moon gave the images a shocking through-line. A convergence, a direction; a goal.

Setrakian felt a surge of energy and excitement. His mind was hunting.

"Ozryel is the angel of death," said Setrakian. "Muslims call him 'he of the four faces, the many eyes, and the many mouths. He of the seventy thousand feet and four thousand wings.' And he has as many eyes and as many tongues as there are men on earth. But you see, that only speaks of how he can multiply, how he can spread . . ."

Fet's thoughts swam. The part that most concerned him was safely extracting the blood worm from Setrakian's jar-sealed vampire heart. The old man had lined the table with battery-powered UV lamps in order to contain the worm. Everything appeared ready, and the jar was close at hand, the fist-size organ throbbing—and yet, now that the time had come, Setrakian was reluctant to butcher the sinister heart.

Setrakian leaned in close to the specimen jar, and a tentacled outgrowth shot out, the mouth-like sucker at its tip adhering to the glass. These blood worms were nasty suckers. Fet understood that the old man had been feeding it drops of his blood for decades now, nursing this ugly thing, and, in doing so, had formed some eerie attachment to it. That was natural enough. But Setrakian's hesitation here contained an emotional component beyond pure melancholy.

This was more like true sorrow. More like despair.

Fet realized something then. Now and then, in the middle of the night, he had seen the old man speaking to the jar, feeding the thing inside. Alone by candlelight he stared at it, whispered to it, and caressed the cold glass containing the unholy flesh. Once Fet swore he'd heard the old man singing to it. Softly, in a foreign tongue—not Armenian—a lullaby . . .

Setrakian had become aware of Fet looking at him. "Forgive me, professor," said Fet.

"But . . . whose **heart** is it? The original story you told us . . ."

Setrakian nodded, having been found out. "Yes . . . that I cut it out of the chest of a young widow in a village in northern Albania? You are right, that tale is not entirely true."

Tears sparkled in the old man's eyes. One drop fell in silence, and, when he finally spoke, he did so in a whisper—as the tale he told required it.

INTERLUDE III

SETRAKIAN'S HEART

ALONG WITH THOUSANDS OF HOLOCAUST SURvivors, Setrakian had arrived in Vienna in 1947, almost entirely penniless, and settled in the Soviet zone of the city. He was able to find some success buying, repairing, and reselling furniture acquired from unclaimed warehouses and estates in all four zones of the city.

One of his clients became also his mentor: Professor Ernst Zelman, one of the few surviving members of the mythical Weiner Kreis, or the Vienna Circle, a turn-of-the-century philosophical society recently dispersed by the Nazis. Zelman had returned to Vienna from exile after having lost most of his family to the Third Reich. He felt enormous empathy with the young Setrakian, and, in a Vienna full of pain and silence—at a time when speaking about "the past" and discussing Nazism was considered abhorrent—

Zelman and Setrakian found great solace in each other's company. Professor Zelman allowed Abraham to borrow freely from his abundant library, and Setrakian, being a bachelor and an insomniac, devoured the books rapidly and systematically. He first applied for studies in philosophy in 1949, and, a few years later, in a very fragmented, very permeable University of Vienna, Abraham Setrakian became associate professor of philosophy.

After he accepted financing from a group headed by Eldritch Palmer, an American industrial magnate with investments in the American zone of Vienna as well as an intense interest in the occult, Setrakian's influence and collection of cultural artifacts expanded at a great rate throughout the early 1960s, capped by his most significant prize, the wolf's-head walking stick of the mysteriously disappeared Jusef Sardu.

But certain developments and revelations out in the field eventually convinced Setrakian that his and Palmer's interests were not compatible. That Palmer's ultimate agenda was, in fact, entirely contrary to Setrakian's intentions to hunt down and expose the vampiric cabal—which led to an ugly rift.

Setrakian knew, beyond doubt, who it was who later spread rumors of his affair with a student, resulting in his removal from the university. The rumors, alas, were entirely true, and Setrakian, freed now by the airing of this secret, swiftly married the lovely Miriam.

Miriam Sacher had survived polio as a child,

and walked with arm and leg braces. To Abraham, she was simply the most exquisite little bird who could not fly. Originally a Romance languages expert, she had enrolled in several of Setrakian's seminars and slowly gained the professor's attention. It was anathema to date a student, so Miriam convinced her wealthy father to hire Abraham as her private tutor. To reach the Sacher family estate, Setrakian had to walk a good hour after taking two trams out of Vienna. The mansion had no electricity, so Abraham and Miriam read by the light of an oil lamp in the family library. Miriam moved around using a wood-and-wicker wheelchair that Setrakian used to push near the bookshelves as new volumes were required. As he did so, he felt the soft, clean scent of Miriam's hair. A scent that intoxicated him and that, as a memory, greatly distracted him in the few hours they spent apart. Soon, their mutual intentions were made manifest and discretion gave way to apprehension as they hid in dark, dusty corners to find each other's breath and saliva.

Disgraced by the university after a prolonged process to remove him from tenure, and facing opposition from Miriam's family, Setrakian the Jew eloped with the blue-blooded Sacher girl and they married in secret in Mönchhof. Only Professor Zelman and a handful of Miriam's friends were in attendance.

As the years went by, Miriam emerged as a partner in his expeditions, a comfort during the dark times, and a true believer in his cause. For over a decade, Setrakian was able to make a living by writing small pamphlets and working as a curator for antique houses all over Europe. Miriam made the most of their modest resources, and nights at the Setrakian house were usually uneventful. Every night, Abraham would rub Miriam's legs with a mixture of alcohol, camphor, and herbs, patiently massaging out the painful knots that cramped muscle and sinew—hiding the fact that, while he did so, his hands hurt as much as her legs. Night after night, the professor told Miriam about ancient knowledge and myth, reciting stories full of hidden meaning and lore. He would end by humming old German lullabies to help her forget her pain and drift into sleep.

In the spring of 1967, Abraham Setrakian picked up Eichhorst's trail in Bulgaria, and a hunger for vengeance against the Nazi rekindled the fire in his belly. Eichhorst, his commandant at Treblinka, was the man who issued Setrakian his craftsman star. He had also twice promised to execute his favorite woodworker, to do so personally. Such was a Jew's lot in the extermination camp.

Setrakian tracked Eichhorst to the Balkans. Albania had been a communist regime since the war, and, for whatever reason, *strigoi* appeared to flourish in similar political and ideological climates. Setrakian had high hopes that his old camp warden—the dark god of that kingdom of industrialized death—might even lead him to the Master.

Because of her physical infirmity, Setrakian left Miriam at a village outside Shkodër, and led a pack horse fifteen kilometers to the ancient town of Drisht. Setrakian pulled the reluctant animal up the steep limestone incline, along old Ottoman paths rising to the hilltop castle.

Drisht Castle (*Kalaja e Drishtit*) dated to the twelfth century, erected as part of a mountaintop chain of Byzantine fortifications. The castle came under Montenegrin and then, briefly, Venetian rule, before the region fell to the Turks in 1478. Now, nearly five hundred years later, the fortress ruins contained a small Muslim village, a small mosque, and the neglected castle, its walls falling prey to nature.

Setrakian discovered the village empty, with little sign of recent activity. The views from the mountaintop out to the Dinaric Alps to the north, and the Adriatic Sea and the Strait of Otranto to the west were sweeping and majestic.

The crumbling stone castle with its centuries of stillness was a spot-on location for vampire hunting. In retrospect, that should have tipped Setrakian off that things were perhaps not as they seemed.

In the belowground chambers, he discovered the coffin. A simple and modern funerary box, a tapered hexagon constructed of all wood, apparently cypress, containing no metal parts, utilizing wooden pegs instead of nails, and leather hinging.

It was not yet nightfall, but the light in the room was not strong enough that he could rely on it to do the job. So Setrakian prepared his silver sword, making ready to dispatch his former tormentor. Weapon set, he raised the lid with his crooked-fingered hand.

The box, indeed, was empty. Emptier than empty: it was bottomless. Fixed to the floor, it functioned as a trapdoor of sorts. Setrakian strapped on a headlamp from his bag and peered down.

The dirt bottomed some fifteen feet below, then tunneled out.

Setrakian loaded himself up with tools—including an extra flashlight, a pouch of batteries, and his long silver knives (his discovery of the killing properties of ultraviolet light in the C range was yet to come—as was the advent of commercially available UV lamps), leaving behind all of his food and most of his water. He tied a rope to the wall chains and lowered himself into the coffin tunnel.

The ammonia smell of *strigoi* discharge was pungent, prompting him to step carefully, to avoid soiling his boots. He made his way through the passages, listening at every turn, picking signal marks into the walls when the tunnel forked, until, after some time, he found he had doubled back to his original marks.

Reconsidering, he decided to retrace his steps and return to the entrance beneath the bottomless coffin. He would climb back out, regroup, and lie in wait for the inhabitants to rise after nightfall.

But when he arrived back at the entrance, looking up, he found that the coffin lid had been shut. And his access rope was gone.

Setrakian had hunted enough *strigoi* that his reaction to this turn of events was not fear but anger. He turned immediately, plunging back into the tunnels with the knowledge that his survival depended upon his being predator and not prey.

He took a different route this time, and eventually encountered a family of four peasant villagers. They were *strigoi*, their red eyes lighting up at his presence, reflected blindly in the beam of his flashlight.

But they were all too weak to attack. The mother was the only one to rise from all fours, Setrakian noticing in her face the characteristic caving of an unnourished vampire: a darkening of the flesh, the articulation of the throat stinger mechanism through the taut skin, and a dazed, somnolent appearance.

He released them—with ease, and without mercy.

He soon encountered two other families, one stronger than the other, but neither able to mount much of a challenge. In another chamber, he found a child *strigoi* who had been destroyed in what appeared to be an ill-fated attempt at vampire cannibalism.

But still, no sign of Eichhorst.

Once he had cleared the ancient cave network of vampires, having discovered no other exit, he returned to the chamber beneath the closed coffin and began chipping away at the ancient stone with his dagger. He hacked out one toehold in the wall, setting to work on another a few feet higher in the opposite wall. As he worked for hours—the silver was a poor choice for the job, cracking and warping, the iron handle and grip proving more useful—he wondered about the wasting village *strigoi* down here. Their presence made little sense. Something was amiss, but Setrakian resisted reasoning it all the way through, pushing down his anxiety in order to focus on the job at hand.

Hours—maybe days—later, out of water and low on batteries, he balanced on the two lower toeholds to carve out the third. His hands were covered with a paste of blood mixed with dust, his tools difficult to hold. Finally, he braced his opposite foot against the sheer wall and reached the lid of the coffin.

With one desperate thrust, he shoved open the top.

He climbed out, emerging paranoid, half-crazed. The pack he had left there was gone, and with it, his extra food and water. Parched, he emerged from the castle into life-saving daylight. The sky was overcast. He had a sense of years having elapsed.

His horse had been slaughtered at the head of the path, gutted, its body cold.

The sky opened over him as he hurried back to the village. A farmer, one he had nodded to on the way up, traded for Setrakian's broken wristwatch some water and rock-hard biscuits, and Setrakian learned, through intensive pantomiming, that he had been underground for three sunsets and three dawns.

He finally returned to the villa he had rented, but Miriam was not there. No note, no nothing—entirely unlike her. He went next door, then across the street. Finally, a man opened his door to him, just a crack.

No, he hadn't seen his wife, the man told him in pidgin Greek.

Setrakian saw a woman cowering behind the man. He asked if something was wrong.

The man explained to him that two children had disappeared from the village the night before. A witch was suspected.

Setrakian returned to his rented villa. He sat heavily in a chair, holding his head in his bloodied, broken hands, and waited for nightfall—for the dark hour of his dear wife's return.

She came to him out of the rain, free of the crutches and braces that had steadied her limbs all her human life. Her hair hung wet, her flesh white and slick, her clothes drenched with mud. She came to him with her head held high, in the manner of a society woman about to welcome a neophyte into her circle of esteem. At her sides stood the two village children she had turned, a boy and a girl still sick with transformation.

Miriam's legs were straight and very dark. Blood had gathered at the lower portion of her extremities and both her hands and feet were now almost entirely black. Gone were her infirm, tentative steps: the atrophied gait which Setrakian had tried nightly to alleviate.

How completely and quickly she had changed from the love of his life into this mad, muddied, glaring creature. Now a *strigoi* with a taste for the children she could not bear in life.

Crying softly, Setrakian rose from his chair, half of him desiring to let it be, to go down into hell with her, to give himself over to vampirism in his despair.

But slay her he did, with much love and many tears. The children he cut down as well, with no regard for their corrupted bodies—though with Miriam, he was determined to preserve a part of her for himself.

Even if one understands that what one is doing is mad, it is indeed still madness—cutting the diseased heart out of one's wife's chest and preserving it, the corrupted organ beating with the craving of a blood worm, inside a pickling jar.

Life is madness, thought Setrakian, done with his butchering, looking about the room. *And so is love.*

The Flatlands

After having a last moment with his late wife's heart, Setrakian uttered something that Fet barely heard and did not understand—it was "Forgive me, dearest"—and then went to work.

He sectioned the heart not with a silver blade, which would have been fatal to the worm, but with a knife of stainless steel—trimming the diseased organ back and back and back. The worm did not make its escape until Setrakian held the heart near one of the UV lamps set around the edge of the table. Thicker than a strand of hair, spindly and quick, the pinkish capillary worm shot out, aiming first for the broken fingers that gripped the knife handle. But Setrakian was much too prepared for that, and it slithered into the center of the table. Setrakian chopped it once with his blade, splitting the worm in two. Fet then trapped the separated ends using two large drinking glasses.

The worms regenerated themselves, exploring the inside rim of their new cages.

Setrakian then set about preparing the experiment. Fet sat back on a stool, watching the worms lash about inside the glass, driven by blood hunger. Fet remembered Setrakian's warning to Eph, about destroying Kelly:

In the act of releasing a loved one . . . you taste what it is to be turned. To go against everything you are. That act changes one forever.

And Nora, about love being the true victim of this plague, the instrument of our downfall:

The undead returning for their Dear Ones. Human love corrupted into vampiric need.

Fet said, "Why didn't they kill you in those tunnels? Since it was a trap?"

Setrakian looked up from his contraption. "Believe it or not, they were afraid of me back then. I was still in the prime of life, I was vital, I was strong. They are indeed sadists, but, you must remember, their numbers were quite small back then. Self-preservation was paramount. Unbridled expansion of their species was a taboo. And yet they had to hurt me. And so they did."

Fet said, "They are still afraid of you."

"Not me. Only what I represent. What I know. In truth, what can one old man do against a horde of vampires?"

Fet did not believe Setrakian's humility, not for a moment.

The old man continued, "I think the fact that we don't give up—this idea that the human spirit keeps going in the face of absolute adversity—puzzles them. They are arrogant. Their origin, if confirmed, will attest to that."

"What is their origin, then?"

"Once we get the book, once I am completely certain . . . I will reveal it to you."

The radio started to fade, and Fet first thought it was his bad ear. He stood and turned the crank, powering the unit, keeping it going. Human voices were largely absent from the airwaves, replaced by heavy interference and occasional high-pitched tones. But one commercial sports radio station still had broadcast power, and though apparently all of its on-air talent were gone, a lone producer remained. He had taken up the microphone, changing the format from Yankees-Mets-Giants-Jets-Rangers-Knicks talk to news updates culled off the Internet and from occasional callers.

". . . the national Web site of the FBI now reports that they have Dr. Ephraim Goodweather in federal custody, following an incident in Brooklyn. He is the fugitive former New York City CDC official who released that first video—remember that? The guy in the shed, chained like a dog. Remember when that demon stuff seemed pretty hysterical and far-fetched? Those were good times. Anyway . . . it says he's been arrested on . . . what's this? Attempted murder? Jeez. Just when you think we might be able to get some real answers. I mean, this guy was at the center of the whole initial thing, if memory serves. Right? He was there at the plane, at Flight 753. And he was wanted for the murder of one of the other first responders, a guy who worked for him, I think the name was Jim Kent. So, clearly, there's something going on with this guy. My opinion—I think they're gonna Oswald him. Two bullets to the gut, and he's silenced forever. Another piece in this giant puzzle that no one seems to be able to put together. Anybody out there has any thoughts on this, any ideas, any theories, and your phone is still working, hit me up on the sports hotline . . ."

Setrakian sat with his eyes closed.

Fet said, "Attempted murder?"

"Palmer," said Setrakian.

"Palmer!" said Fet. "You mean—it's not some bogus charge?" Fet's shock quickly turned to appreciation. "Gunning down Palmer. Christ. Good ol' doc. Why didn't I think of that?"

"I am very glad you did not."

Fet ran his fingers through the hair on the top of his head, as though waking himself up. "And then there were two, huh?" He stepped back, looking out through the half-open door to the storefront. Dusk was falling through the windows beyond. "So you knew about this?"

"I suspected."

"You didn't want to stop him?"

"I could see—there was no stopping. A man has to act on his own impulses sometimes. Understand—he is a medical scientist caught up in a pandemic, the source of which defies everything he thought he knew. Add to that the personal conflict involving his wife. He took the course he thought was right."

"Bold move. Would it have meant anything? If he had succeeded?"

"Oh, I think so." Setrakian went back to his tinkering.

Fet smiled. "I didn't think he had it in him."

"I'm sure he didn't either."

Fet thought he saw a shadow pass before the front windows then. He had been half-turned away, the image in his periphery. It had struck him as a large being.

"I think we've got a customer," said Fet, hurrying to the back door.

Setrakian stood, reaching quickly for his wolf's-head staff, twisting the top and exposing a few inches of silver.

"Stay," said Fet. "Be ready." He took his loaded nail gun and a sword, and slipped out the back door, fearing the arrival of the Master.

Out on the back curb, as soon as he closed the door, Fet saw the big man. Thick-browed, a hulking man in his sixties, as big as Fet. He stood with a slight crouch, favoring one leg. His open hands were out, resembling a wrestler's stance.

Not the Master. Not even a vampire. The man's eyes confirmed it. Even newly turned vampires move strangely, less like a human and more like an animal, or a bug.

Two others stepped from behind the DPW van. One was all silvered up with jewelry, short and wide and powerful-looking, snarling like a junkyard dog larded with bling. The other was younger, holding the tip of a long sword out toward Fet, aimed at his throat.

So they knew their silver. "I'm human," said Fet. "You guys are looking to loot something, I got nothing here but rat poison."

"We are looking for an old man," came a voice behind Fet. He turned, keeping all comers in front of him. The new one was Gus, his torn shirt collar partially revealing the phrase SOY COMO SOY tattooed across his clavicle. He carried a long silver knife in his hand.

Three Mexican gangbangers and an old ex-wrestler with hands the size of thick steaks. "It's getting dark, boys," said Fet. "You should be moving right along."

Creem, the silver-knuckled one, said, "Now what?"

Gus said to Fet, "The pawnbroker. Where is he?"

Fet held pat. These punks packed slaying weapons, but he didn't know them, and what he didn't know he didn't like. "Don't know who you're talking about."

Gus wasn't buying. "I guess we go door to door, then, motherfucker."

Fet said, "You do, you're gonna have to go through me." He pointed with his nail gun. "And just so you know—this baby right here is nasty. The nail just fastens to the bone. Homes right in on it. Vampire or not, damage will be done. I'll hear you squeal when you try to pry a couple of silvery inches out of your fucking eye socket, *cholo*."

"Vasiliy," said Setrakian, exiting out the back door, staff in hand.

Gus saw him, saw the old man's hands. All busted up, just as he remembered. The pawnbroker looked even older now, smaller. It had been years since they'd met a few weeks ago. He straightened, uncertain if the old man would recognize him.

Setrakian looked him over. "From the jail."

Fet said, "Jail?"

Setrakian reached out and patted Gus's arm familiarly. "You listened. You learned. And you survived."

"*A guevo.* I survived. And you—you got out."

"I had a stroke of good fortune," said Setrakian. He looked at the others. "But what of your friend? The sick one. You did what you had to do?"

Gus winced, remembering. "*Si.* I did what I had to do. And I've been fucking doing it ever since."

Angel dug into a knapsack on his shoulder, and Fet readied his nail gun. "Easy, big bear," he said.

Angel pulled out the silver case recovered from the pawnshop. Gus went and took it from him, opening it, removing the card inside, and handing it to the pawnbroker.

It contained Fet's address.

Setrakian noticed that the case was dented and blackened, one corner warped from heat.

Gus told him, "They sent a crew for you. Used smoke cover to attack in daytime. They were all over your shop when we got there." Gus nodded to the others. "We had to blow up your place to get out of there with our blood still red."

Setrakian showed only a flicker of regret, passing quickly. "So—you have joined the fight."

"Who, me?" said Gus, brandishing his silver blade. "I am the fight. Been flushing 'em out these past few days—way too many to count."

Setrakian looked more closely at Gus's weapon, showing concern. "Where, may I ask, did you get such well-made arms?"

"From the fucking source," said Gus. "They came for me when I was still in handcuffs, running from the law. Pulled me right off the street."

Setrakian's expression turned dark. "Who are 'they'?"

"Them. The old ones."

Setrakian said, "The Ancients."

"Holy Jesus," said Fet.

Setrakian motioned to him to be patient. "Please," he said to Gus. "Explain."

Gus did so, recounting the Ancients' offer, that they were holding his mother, and how he had recruited the Sapphires out of Jersey City to work at his side as day hunters.

"Mercenaries," said Setrakian.

Gus took that as a compliment. "We're mopping the floor with milk blood. A tight hit squad, good vampire killers. Vampire shit-kickers, more like it."

Angel nodded. He liked this kid.

"The Ancients," Gus said. "They feel that this is all a concerted attack. Breaking their breeding rules, risking exposure. Shock and Awe, I guess . . ."

Fet coughed out a laugh. "You guess? You're joking. No? You fucking dropout assassins have no idea what's going down here. You don't even know whose side you're really on."

"Hold, please." Setrakian silenced Fet with a hand, thinking. "Do they know that you have come to me?"

"No," said Gus.

"They will soon. And they will not be pleased." Setrakian put up his hands, reassuring the confused Gus. "Fret not. It is all a big mess, a bad situation for anyone with red blood in their veins. I am very glad you sought me out again."

Fet had learned to like the brightness that came into the old man's eyes when he was getting an idea. It helped Fet relax a little.

Setrakian said to Gus, "I think perhaps there is something you can do for me."

Gus shot a cutting look at Fet, as though saying, *Take that*. "Name it," he said to Setrakian. "I owe you plenty."

"You will take my friend and me to the Ancients."

Brooklyn-Queens FBI Resident Agency

EPH SAT ALONE in the debriefing room, his elbows on a scratched table, calmly rubbing at his hands. The room smelled of old coffee, though there was none present. The ceiling-lamp light fell on the one-way mirror, illuminating a single human handprint, the ghostly remnant of a recent interrogation.

Strange knowing you are being watched, even studied. It affected what you do, down to your very posture, the way you licked your lips, how you looked at or didn't look at yourself in the mirror, behind which lurked your captors. If lab rats knew their behavior was being scrutinized, then every maze-and-cheese experiment would take on an extra dimension.

Eph looked forward to their questions, perhaps more than the FBI was looking forward to his answers. He hoped that their inquiries would give him a sense of the investigation at hand, and, in doing so, let him know to what extent the vampire invasion was currently understood by law enforcement and the powers that be.

He had once read that falling asleep while awaiting questioning is a leading indicator of a suspect's culpability. The reason was something about how the lack of a physical outlet for one's anxiety exhausted the guilty mind—that, coupled with an unconscious need to hide or escape.

Eph was plenty tired, and sore, but more than that, he felt relief. He was done. Under arrest, in federal custody. No more fight, no more struggle. He was of little use to Setrakian and Fet anyway. With Zack and Nora now safely out of the hot zone, speeding south to Harrisburg, it seemed to him that sitting here in the penalty box was preferable to warming the bench.

Two agents entered without introduction. They handcuffed his wrists, Eph thinking that strange. They cuffed them not behind his back but in front of him, then pulled him out of the chair and walked him from the room.

They led him past the mostly empty bullpen to a key-access elevator. No one said anything on the ride up. The door opened on an unadorned access hallway, which they followed to a short flight of stairs, leading to a door to the roof.

A helicopter was parked there, its rotors already speeding up, chopping into the night air. Too noisy to ask questions, so Eph crouch-walked with the other two into the belly of the bird, and sat while they seat-belted him in.

The chopper lifted off, rising over Kew Gardens and greater Brooklyn. Eph saw the blocks burning, the helicopter weaving between great plumes of thick, black smoke. All this devastation raging below him. *Surreal* didn't begin to describe it.

He realized they were crossing the East River, and then really wondered where they were taking him. He saw the police and fire lights spinning on the Brooklyn Bridge, but no moving cars, no people. Lower Manhattan came up fast around them, the helicopter dipping lower, the tallest buildings limiting his view.

Eph knew that the FBI headquarters were in Federal Plaza, a few blocks north of City Hall. But no, they remained close to the Financial District.

The chopper climbed again, zeroing in on the only lit rooftop for blocks around: a red ring of safety lights demarking a helipad. The bird touched down gently, and the agents unbuckled Eph's seat belt. They got him up out of his seat without getting up themselves, essentially kicking him to the rooftop.

He remained in a standing crouch, air whipping at his clothes as the bird lifted off again, turning in the air and whirring away, back toward Brooklyn. Leaving him alone—and still handcuffed.

Eph smelled burning and ocean salt, the troposphere over Manhattan clogged with smoke. He remembered how the dust trail of the World Trade Center—white-gray, that—rose and flattened once it reached a certain elevation, then spread out over the skyline in a cloud of despair.

This cloud was black, blocking out the stars, making a dark night even darker.

He turned in a circle, bewildered. He walked beyond the ring of red landing lights, and, around one of the giant air-conditioning units, saw an open door, faint light emanating from within. He walked to it, stopping there with his cuffed hands outstretched, debating whether or not to go inside, then realizing that he had no choice. It was either sprout wings or see this thing through.

Faint red light inside came from an EXIT sign. A long staircase led down to another propped-open door. Through it was a carpeted hallway with expensive accent lighting. A man dressed in a dark suit stood halfway down, hands folded at his waist. Eph stopped, ready to run.

The man said nothing. He did nothing. Eph could see that he was human, not vampire.

Next to him, built into the wall, was a logo depicting a black orb bisected by a steel-blue line.

The corporate symbol for the Stoneheart Group. Eph realized, for the first time, that it resembled the occulted sun winking its eye closed.

His adrenaline kicked in, his body preparing to fight. But the Stoneheart man turned and walked away to the end of the hall, to a door, which he opened and held.

Eph walked toward him, warily, sliding past the man and through the door. The man did not follow, instead closing the door with him remaining on the other side.

Art adorned the walls of the vast room, super-sized canvases depicting nightmarish imagery and violent abstraction. Music played faintly, seeming to find his ears in the same measured volume as he moved throughout the room.

Around a corner, at the edge of the building walled in glass, looking north at the suffering island of Manhattan, was a table set for one.

A stream of low light spilled down onto the white linen, making it glow. A butler, or a waiter—a servant of some kind—arrived when Eph did, pulling out the only chair for him. Eph looked at the man—he was old, a domestic for life—the servant watching him without meeting his eye, standing with every expectation that his guest should take the seat offered him.

And so Eph did. The chair was pushed in beneath the table, a napkin opened and laid across his right thigh, and then the servant walked away.

Eph looked at the great windows. The reflection made it appear he was seated outside, at a table hovering some seventy-eight stories over Manhattan, while the city roiled in paroxysms of violence beneath him.

A slight whirring noise undercut the pleasant symphony. A motorized wheelchair appeared out of the gloom, and Eldritch Palmer, his frail hand operating the steering stick, rolled across the polished floor to the opposite side of the table.

Eph began to get to his feet—but then Mr. Fitzwilliam, Palmer's bodyguard-cum-nurse, appeared in the shadows. The guy was bulging out of his suit, his orange hair cut high and tight, like a small, contained fire atop his boulder of a head.

Eph relented, sitting back down.

Palmer pulled in so that the front of his chair arms lined up with the tabletop. Once he was set, he looked across at Eph. Palmer's head resembled a triangle: broad-crowned with S-shaped veins evident at both temples, narrowing to a chin that trembled with age.

"You are a terrible shot, Dr. Goodweather," said Palmer. "Killing me might have impeded our progress somewhat, but only temporarily. However, you caused irreversible liver damage to one of my bodyguards. Not very hero-like, I must say."

Eph said nothing, still stunned by this sudden change of venue from the FBI in Brooklyn to Palmer's Wall Street penthouse.

Palmer said, "Setrakian sent you to kill me, did he not?"

Eph said, "He did not. In fact, in his own way, I think he tried to talk me out of it. I went on my own."

Palmer frowned, disappointed. "I must admit, I wish he was here, rather than you. Someone who could relate to what I have done, at least. The scope of my achievement. Someone who would understand the magnitude of my deeds, even as he condemned them." Palmer signaled to Mr. Fitzwilliam. "Setrakian is not the man you think he is," said Palmer.

"No?" said Eph. "Who do I think he is?"

Mr. Fitzwilliam approached, pulling a large piece of medical equipment on casters, a machine with whose function Eph was not familiar.

Palmer said, "You see him as the kindly old man, the white wizard. The humble genius."

Eph said nothing as Mr. Fitzwilliam pulled up Palmer's shirt, revealing twin valves implanted in his thin side, the man's flesh hashed with scars. Mr. Fitzwilliam connected two tubes from the machine to the valves, taping them sealed, then switched on the machine. A feeder of some kind.

Palmer said, "In fact, he is a blunderer. A butcher, a psychopath, and a disgraced scholar. A failure in every respect."

Palmer's words made Eph smile. "If he was such a failure, you wouldn't be talking about him now, wishing I were him."

Palmer blinked sleepily. He raised his hand again and a distant door opened, a figure emerging. Eph braced himself, wondering what Palmer had in store for him—if this scallywag had a taste for revenge—but it was only the servant again, this time carrying a small tray on his fingertips.

He swept in front of Eph and set a cocktail

down before him, rocks of ice floating in amber fluid.

Palmer said, "I am told you are a man who enjoys a stiff drink."

Eph looked at the drink, then back at Palmer. "What is this?"

"A Manhattan," said Palmer. "It seemed appropriate."

"Not the damn drink. Why am I here?"

"You are my guest for dinner. A last meal. Not yours—mine." He nodded to the machine feeding him.

The servant returned with a plate covered with a stainless-steel dome. He set it in front of Eph and removed the cover. Glazed black cod, baby potatoes, Oriental vegetable medley—all warm and steaming.

Eph didn't move, looking down at it.

"Come now, Dr. Goodweather. You haven't seen food like this in days. And don't worry about it having been tampered with, poisoned or drugged. If I wanted you dead, Mr. Fitzwilliam here would see to it promptly and then enjoy your meal himself."

Eph had actually been looking at the utensils set out for him. He grasped the sterling-silver knife, holding it up so that it caught the light.

"Silver, yes," said Palmer. "No vampires here tonight."

Eph took up his fork and, with his eyes on Palmer, and his handcuffs clinking, cut into the fish. Palmer watched as he brought a morsel to his mouth, chewing it, juices exploding on his dry tongue, his belly rumbling with anticipation.

"It has been decades since I ingested food orally," said Palmer. "I grew accustomed to not eating while recuperating from various surgical procedures. Really, you can lose your taste for food surprisingly easily."

He watched Eph chew and swallow.

"After a time, the simple act of eating comes to appear quite animalistic. Grotesque, in fact. No different than a cat consuming a dead bird. The mouth-throat-stomach digestive tract is such a crude path to nourishment. So primitive."

Eph said, "We're all just animals to you, is that it?"

" 'Customers' is the accepted term. But certainly. We, the overclass, have taken those basic human drives and advanced our own selves through their exploitation. We have monetized human consumption, manipulated morals and laws to direct the masses by fear or hatred, and, in doing so, have managed to create a system of wealth and remuneration that has concentrated the vast majority of the world's wealth in the hands of a select few. Over the course of two thousand years, I believe this system worked pretty well. But all good things must end. You saw, with the recent market crash, how we have been building to this impossible end. Money built upon money built upon money. Two choices remain. Either utter collapse, which appeals to no one, or the richest push the pedal to the floor and take it all. And here we are now."

Eph said, "You brought the Master here. You arranged for him to be on that airplane."

"Indeed. But, doctor, I have been so consumed with the orchestration of this endeavor for lo these past ten years that to recount it all for you now would truly be a waste of my last hours. If you don't mind."

"You are selling out the human race so you can live forever—as a vampire?"

Palmer put his hands together in a gesture of prayer, but only to rub his palms and generate some warmth. "Are you aware that this very island was once home to as many different species as Yellowstone National Park?"

"No, I wasn't. So we humans had it coming, is that your point?"

Palmer laughed softly. "No, no. No, that is not it. Far too moralistic. Any dominant species would have ravaged the land with equal or grander enthusiasm. My point is that the land doesn't care. The sky doesn't care. The planet doesn't care. The entire system is structured around a long-winded decay and an eventual rebirth. Why are you so precious about humanity? You can already feel it slipping away from you now. You're falling apart. Is the sensation really all that bad?"

Eph remembered—with a spike of shame now—his apathy in the FBI debriefing room after his arrest. He looked with disgust at the cocktail Palmer expected him to drink.

Palmer continued, "The smart move would have been to cut a deal."

Eph said, "I had nothing to offer."

Palmer considered this. "Is that why you still resist?"

"Partly. Why should people like you have all the fun?"

Palmer's hands returned to his armrests with the certainty of revelation. "It's the myths, isn't it? Movies and books and fables. It has become ingrained. The entertainment we sold, that was meant to placate you. To keep you down but still dreaming. Keep you wanting. Hoping. Coveting. Anything to direct your attention away from your sense of the animal, toward the fiction of a greater existence—a higher purpose." He smiled again. "Something beyond the cycle of birth, re-production, death."

Eph pointed at Palmer with his fork. "But isn't that what you're doing now? You think you are about to go beyond death. You believe in the same fictions."

"Me? A victim of the same great myth?" Palmer considered this angle, then discounted it. "I have made a new fate. I am forsaking death for deliverance. My point is—this humanity your heart bleeds for is already subservient, and fully programmed for subjugation."

Eph looked up. "Subjugation? What do you mean by that?"

Palmer shook his head. "I am not about to detail everything for you. Not because you might do something heroic with this information—you cannot. It is too late. The die is already cast."

Eph's mind reeled. He remembered Palmer's speech from earlier in the day, his testimony. "Why do you want a quarantine now? Sealing off cities? What is the point? Unless . . . are you trying to herd us together?"

Palmer did not answer.

Eph went on, "They can't turn everybody, because then there would be no blood meals. You need a reliable food source." It hit him then, what Palmer had said. "Food delivery. The meatpacking plants. Are you . . . ? No . . ."

Palmer folded his old hands in his lap.

Eph pressed him. "And then—what about the nuclear power plants? Why do you need them to come on line?"

Palmer answered by saying again, "The die is already cast."

Eph set down his fork, swiping the knife blade with his napkin before setting it down as well. These revelations had killed his body's junkie-like urge for protein.

"You're not insane," said Eph, actively trying to read him now. "You're not even evil. You are desperate, and certainly megalomaniacal. Absolutely perverse. Is all this spun out of a rich man's fear of death? You trying to buy your way out of it? Actually choosing the alternative? But—for what? What have you *not* already done that you lust after? What will be left for you to lust for?"

For the briefest moment, Palmer's eyes showed a hint of fragility, perhaps even fear. In that instant he was revealed to be just what he was: a fragile, sick old man.

"You don't understand, Dr. Goodweather. I have been sick all my life. *All my life.* I had no childhood. No adolescence. I have been fighting against my own rot for as long as I can remember. Fear death? I walk with it every day. What I want now is to transcend it. To silence it. For what has being human ever done for me? Every pleasure I have ever experienced has been tainted by the whisper of decay and disease."

"But—to be a vampire? A . . . a creature? A bloodsucking thing?"

"Well . . . arrangements have been made. I will be exalted somewhat. Even at the next stage, there has to be a class system, you know. And I have been promised a seat at the very top."

"Promised by a vampire. A virus. What about *his* will? He is going to invade yours as he has all the others—possess it, make yours an extension of his own. What good is that? Merely trading one whisper for another . . ."

"I have dealt with worse, believe me. But it is kind of you to show such concern for my well-being." Palmer looked to the great windows, beyond their reflection to the dying city below. "People will prefer any fate to this. They will welcome our alternative. You'll see. They will accept any system, any order, that promises them the illusion of security." He looked back. "But you haven't touched your drink."

Eph said, "Maybe I'm not so preprogrammed. Maybe people are more unpredictable than you think."

"I don't think so. Every model has its individual anomalies. A renowned doctor and scientist becomes an assassin. Amusing. What most people lack is vision—a vision of the truth. The ability to act with deadly certainty. No, as a group—a *herd*, that is your word—they are easily led, and wonderfully predictable. Capable of selling, turning, killing those that they profess to love in exchange for peace of mind or a scrap of food." Palmer shrugged, disappointed that Eph was evidently through eating and the meal was over. "You will be going back to the FBI now."

"Those agents are in on it? How big is this conspiracy?"

"'Those agents'?" Palmer shook his head. "As with any bureaucratic institution—say, for instance, the CDC—once you seize control of the top, the rest of the organization simply follows orders. The Ancients have operated that way for years. The Master is no exception. Don't you see that this is why governments were established in the first place? So, no, there is no conspiracy, Dr. Goodweather. This is the very same structure that has existed since the beginning of recorded time."

Mr. Fitzwilliam unplugged Palmer from his feeding machine. Eph saw that Palmer was already half a vampire; that the jump from intravenous nourishment to a blood meal was not a great one. "Why did you have me here?"

"Not to gloat. I believe that has been made clear. Nor to unburden my soul." Palmer chuckled before returning to seriousness. "This is my last night as a man. Dinner with my would-be assassin struck me as a meaningful part of the program. Tomorrow, Dr. Goodweather, I will exist in a place beyond death's reach. And your kind will exist—"

"My kind?" said Eph, interrupting.

"Your kind will exist in a manner beyond all hope. I have delivered to you a new Messiah, and the reckoning is at hand. The mythmakers were right, save for their characterization of the second coming of a Messiah. He will indeed raise the dead. He will preside over the final judgment. God promises eternal life. The Master delivers it. And he will establish his kingdom on earth."

"And what does that make *you*? The king-maker? It sounds to me like you are one more drone doing his bidding."

Palmer pursed his dry lips in a condescending manner. "I see. Another clumsy attempt to instill doubt in me. Dr. Barnes warned me against your stubbornness. But I suppose you have to try again and again—"

"I'm not trying anything. If you can't see that he's been stringing you along, then you deserve to get it in the neck."

Palmer held his expression steady. What worked behind it—that was another matter. "Tomorrow," he said, "is the day."

"And why would he deign to share power with another?" said Eph. He sat up, his hands dropping below the table. He was winging it here, but it felt right. "Think about it. What sort of contract is holding him to this arrangement? What'd you two do, shake hands? You're not blood brothers— not yet. Best-case scenario, by this time tomorrow you'll be just another bloodsucker in the hive. Take it from an epidemiologist. Viruses don't make deals."

"He would be nowhere without me."

"Without your money. Without your mundane influence, yes. All of which"—Eph nodded at the anarchy below them—"exist no more."

Mr. Fitzwilliam stepped forward then, moving to Eph's side. "The helicopter has returned."

"And so it is good evening, Dr. Goodweather," said Palmer, wheeling back from the table. "And good-bye."

"He's been out there turning folks for free, left and right. So ask yourself this. If you're so damn important, Palmer—why make you wait in line?"

Palmer was rolling slowly away. Mr. Fitzwilliam hoisted Eph roughly to his feet. Eph was lucky: the silver knife he had hidden, tucked inside his waistband, only grazed his upper thigh.

"What's in it for you?" Eph asked Mr. Fitzwilliam. "You're too healthy to be dreaming of eternal life as a bloodsucker."

Mr. Fitzwilliam said nothing. The weapon remained tight against Eph's hip as he was led away, back up to the roof.

RAINFALL

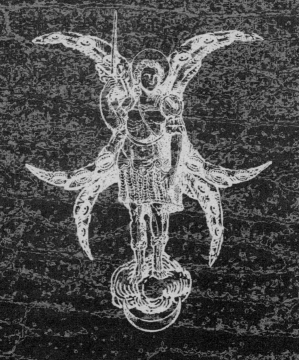

THUD-BUMP!

Nora shivered at the first impact. Everyone felt it, but few realized what it was. She didn't know much herself about the North River Tunnels that connected Manhattan and New Jersey. She guessed that, under normal circumstances—which, let's face it, didn't exist anymore—it was maybe a two-to-three-minute trip total, traveling deep below the Hudson River. A one-way trip, no stopping. The only way in or out through the surface entrance and exit. They probably hadn't even hit the half-way point, the deepest part, yet.

Bam-BAMM-bam-bam-bam.

Another hit, and the sound and vibration of grinding beneath the train's chassis. The noise traveling from the front, bumping beneath her feet all the way to the back of the train, and gone. Her father, driving her uncle's Cadillac many years ago, once ran over a big badger driving through the Adirondacks; this noise was almost the same, only bigger.

This was no badger.

Nor, she suspected, was it human.

Dread enveloped her. The thumping roused her mother, and Nora instinctively grabbed her frail hand. In response, she got a vague smile and a vacant stare.

Better that way, thought Nora, with an extra chill. Better not to deal with her questions, her suspicions, her fears. Nora had plenty of her own.

Zack remained under the influence of his earbuds, eyes closed, head bobbing gently over the backpack on his lap—grooving or maybe dozing. Either way, he was unaware of the bumps and the sense of concern growing in their train car. Though not for long . . .

Bump-CRUNCH.

A gasp went up. Impacts more frequent now, the noises louder. Nora prayed they would get through the tunnel in time. The one thing she had always hated about trains and subways: you can never see out the front windows. You don't see what the driver sees. All you get is a blur. You never see what's coming.

More hits. She thought she could distinguish the cracking of bones and—another!—an inhuman squeal, not unlike a pig.

The conductor evidently had had enough. The emergency brakes engaged with a metallic screech, grating like steel fingernails against the chalkboard of Nora's fear.

Standing passengers grabbed seatbacks and overhead racks. The bumping slowed and became agonizingly more pronounced, the weight of the train crushing bodies beneath them. Zack's head came up and his eyes opened and he looked at Nora.

The train went into a skid, its wheels screaming—then a great shudder and the interior compartment shook with a violence that threw people to the ground.

The train shrieked to a stop, the car tilted to the right.

They had jumped the track.

Derailed.

Lights inside the train flickered and died. A groan went up, with notes of panic.

Then emergency lights came on, but pale.

Nora pulled Zack to his feet. Time to get moving. She pulled her mother with her, starting toward the front of the car before everyone else on the train had recovered. She wanted to get a look at the tunnel by the train's headlight. But she saw immediately that way was impassable. Too many people, too much thrown luggage.

Nora tugged on the strap of the weapon bag across her chest and pushed them the other way, toward the exit between cars. She was playing nice, waiting for fellow passengers to get their bags, when she heard the screaming start in the first car.

Every head turned.

Nora said, "Come on!" She pulled on them both, shoving her way through bodies toward the exits. Let the other people look; she had two lives to protect, never mind her own.

At the end of the car, waiting for some guy to pry open the automatic doors, Nora glanced back behind her.

Over the heads of the confused passengers, she saw frenzied movement in the next car . . . dark figures moving quickly . . . and then a burst of arterial blood spraying against the glass door separating compartments.

G us and his crew had been outfitted by the hunters with armor-plated Hummers, black with chrome accents. Most of the chrome was gone now, due to the fact that, in order to get across bridges and up city streets, you had to do some contact driving.

Gus was heading the wrong way across 59th Street, his headlamps the only lights on the road. Fet sat up front, because of his size. The weapon bag was at his feet. Angel and the others were in another vehicle.

The radio was on, the sports talk host having racked some music in order to give his voice or maybe his bladder a break. Fet realized, as Gus cut hard up onto the sidewalk in order to avoid a knot of abandoned vehicles, that the song was Elton John's "Don't Let the Sun Go Down on Me."

He snapped off the radio, saying, "That's not funny."

They pulled up fast, at the foot of a building overlooking Central Park, exactly the sort of place where Fet always imagined a vampire would reside. Seen from the sidewalk below, it was outlined against the smoky sky like a gothic tower.

Fet entered the front door with Setrakian at his side, both men carrying their swords. Angel trailed them, Gus whistling a tune next to him.

The lobby of rich brown wallpaper was dimly lit and empty. Gus had a key that operated the passenger elevator, a small cage of green iron, its lift cables visible, Victorian styling inside and out.

The top-floor hallway was under construction, or at least left to appear that way. Gus laid his weapons down atop a table-like length of scaffolding. "Everybody disarm here," he said.

Fet looked at Setrakian. Setrakian made no move to relinquish his staff, so Fet kept a tight hold on his sword.

"Fine, have it your way," said Gus.

Angel remained behind as Gus led them inside the only door, up three steps into a dark anteroom. There was the usual light tincture of ammonia and earth, and a sensation of heat not artificially manufactured. Gus parted a heavy curtain, revealing a wide room with three windows overlooking the park.

Silhouetted before each window were three beings, hairless, unclothed, standing as still as the building itself, arranged like statues standing guard over the canyon of Central Park.

Fet raised his silver sword, the blade angling

upward like the needle of a gauge measuring the presence of evil. All at once, he felt his hand struck, the sword handle springing loose from his grip. His other arm, the one gripping the weapon bag, jumped at the shoulder, suddenly lighter.

The bag handles had been cut. He turned his head in time to see his blade enter the side wall, piercing it deeply, quivering, the bag of weapons dangling from it.

He then felt a knife at the side of his throat. Not a silver blade, but instead the point of a long iron spike.

A face, next to him—so pale, it glowed. Its eyes bore the deep red of vampiric possession, its mouth curled into a toothless scowl. Its swollen throat pulsed, not with blood flow but anticipation.

"Hey . . ." said Fet, his voice disappearing into nothingness.

He was done for. The speed with which these ones moved was incredible. So much faster than the animals outside.

But the three beings at the windows—they had not moved.

Setrakian.

The voice, appearing within his mind, was accompanied by a numbing sensation that had the effect of clouding his thoughts.

Fet tried to look over at the old professor. He still held his staff, the interior blade sheathed. Another hunter stood at his side, holding a similar spike to his temple.

Gus walked past them. He said, "They're with me."

They are silver-armed. A hunter's voice—not as debilitating as the other.

Setrakian said, "I come not to destroy you. Not this time."

You would never get so close.

"But I have been close in the past, and you know it. Let us not rehash old battles. I wish to set all that aside for the time being. I have placed myself at your mercy for a reason. I want to deal."

To deal? What could you possibly have to offer?

"The book. And the Master."

Fet felt the vampire goon ease off his neck just a few millimeters, the point of the spike still in contact with his flesh but no longer poking at his throat.

The beings at the windows never moved, the commanding voice in his head unwavering.

And what is it you want in return?

Setrakian said, "The world."

Nora spotted the dark figures siphoning passengers in the aft car. She kicked at the back of the knee of the man in front of her, pulling her mother and Zack past him, shouldering aside a woman in a business suit and sneakers in order to exit the derailed train.

Somehow, she got her mother down the long step without dropping her. Nora looked forward to where the front car had left the track, angled tight against the tunnel wall, and realized she had to go the other way.

She had departed the claustrophobia of the stuck train for the claustrophobia of an under-river tunnel.

Nora unzipped the side compartment on her travel duffel and pulled out her Luma lamp. She powered it on, the battery humming to life, the UVC bulb crackling indigo, burning hot.

The tracks lit up before her. Vampire discharge was everywhere, fluorescent guano, covering the floor and sprayed on the walls. Evidently, they had been crossing this way to the mainland for days, and by the thousands. It was the perfect environment for them: dark, dirty, and concealed from surface eyes.

Others disembarked behind them, a few using mobile phone screens to light their way. "Oh, my God!" one shrieked.

Nora turned and saw, by the light of the passengers' phones, the train wheels goopy with white vampire blood. Gobs of pale skin and the black gristle of crushed bones hung from the undercarriage. Nora wondered if they were run down accidentally—or had they thrown themselves in the path of the charging train?

Thrown themselves seemed most likely. And if so—then what for?

Nora thought she knew. With the image of Kelly still bright in her mind, Nora threw one arm around Zack, taking her mother by the hand and running for the rear of the train.

New Jersey was a long walk away, and they were not alone here.

They heard screaming aboard the train now. Passengers being mauled by pale creatures marauding through the cars. Nora tried to keep Zack from looking up and seeing the faces pressed against the windows, regurgitating saliva and blood.

Nora got to the end of the train, rounding it—stepping over crushed vampire corpses on the tracks, using her UV light to kill any lurking blood worms—and starting up the other side, where there was a clear path toward the front car.

Tunnels carry and distort noises. Nora wasn't sure what she was hearing, but its presence put an extra scare into her. She exhorted the people following them to stop a moment and be quiet and still.

She heard a noise like scuttling, only many times repeated and magnified through the tunnel. Coming behind them, in the same direction the train had been traveling. A horde of footsteps.

The light from the cell phone screens and Nora's UV lamp had very little range. Something was coming at them out of the dark void, and Nora corralled Zack and her mother and started running the other way.

The hunter pulled back from Fet's side, his spike still poised at Fet's neck. Setrakian had started to tell the Ancients about Eldritch Palmer's association with the Master.

We know already. He came to us some time ago, petitioning us for immortality.

"And you refused him. So he went across the street."

He did not meet our criteria. Eternity is a beautiful gift, entrance into an immortal aristocracy. We are rigorously selective.

The voice reverberating inside Fet's head sounded like a scolding parent's multiplied a thousandfold. He looked at the hunter next to him and wondered: some long-dead European king? Alexander the Great? Howard Hughes?

No—not these hunters. Fet guessed he was an elite soldier in his former life. Plucked off a battlefield, perhaps during a special-ops mission. Drafted by the ultimate selective service. But who knew which army? What era? Vietnam? Normandy? Thermopylae?

Setrakian said—confirming for himself lifelong theories as he stated these facts—"The Ancients are connected to the human world at its uppermost levels. They assume the initiate's wealth, which helps them insulate themselves and assert their influence across the globe."

Were it a simple business transaction, his wealth is substantial enough. But we require more than riches. What we seek is power, access, and obedience. He lacked the last.

"Palmer grew angry when the gift was refused him. So he sought out the rogue Master, the young one—"

You seek to know all, Setrakian. Greedy until the end. Let us agree that you are half-correct in every-

thing. Palmer may have sought out the Seventh, yes. But be assured—it was the Seventh who found him.

"Do you know what it is he wants?"

We do know.

"You must know then that you are in trouble. The Master is creating minions by the thousands, too many for your hunters to cut down. His strain is spreading. These are beings you cannot control, not through power or influence."

You spoke of the Silver Codex.

The power of their voices made Fet squint.

Setrakian stepped forward. "What I want from you is unlimited financial support. I require it immediately."

The auction. Don't you think we have considered this before?

"But bidding on it yourselves, employing a human representative, risked exposure. Impossible to guarantee the motives. Better to scuttle each potential sale throughout the years. But that will not be possible this time. I am certain that the timing of this widespread attack, the occultation of the Earth, and the reappearance of the book are no coincidence. It is all aligned. Do you deny this cosmic symmetry?"

We do not. But then again, the outcome will follow the design no matter what we do.

"Doing nothing seems to me like a flawed plan."

And what would you want in return?

"A brief glimpse at its contents. Handcrafted in silver, this book is the one human creation you cannot possess. I have seen the Silver Codex, as you refer to it. It holds many revelations, I can guarantee you that. You would be wise to see what mankind knows of your origin."

Half-truths and speculation.

"Is it? Can you take that chance? Mal'akh Elohim?"

A pause. Fet felt his head relax a moment. He could have sworn he saw the Ancient purse its lips in disgust.

Unlikely alliances are often the most productive.

"Let me be quite clear here. I offer you no alliance. This is nothing more than a wartime truce. The enemy of my enemy is in this instance neither my friend nor yours. I promise nothing other than a viewing of the book, and through it, a chance to defeat the rogue Master before he destroys you. But once this agreement is consummated, I promise you only that the fight will continue. I will come after you again. And you after me . . ."

Once you view the book, Setrakian, we cannot allow you to live. You must know that. This holds for any human.

Fet swallowed and said, "I'm not much of a reader anyway . . ."

Setrakian said, "I accept. And now that we understand each other, there is one other thing I need. Not from you, but from your man here. From Gus."

Gus stepped in front of the old man and Fet. "Just so long as it involves killing."

* * *

There was no ribbon-cutting ceremony. No giant pair of prop scissors, no dignitaries or politicians. No fanfare at all.

The Locust Valley Nuclear Power Plant went online at 5:23 A.M. Resident Nuclear Regulatory Commission inspectors oversaw the procedures from the control room of the $17 billion facility.

Locust Valley was a nuclear fission facility, operating twin thermal, light-water-moderated Generation III reactors. All site and safety reviews had been completed before the Uranium-235 bundles and the control rods were introduced into the water inside the pressurized core.

The principle of controlled fission is likened to a nuclear bomb exploding at a slow, steady rate, rather than a millisecond. The heat produced generates electricity, which is then harnessed and delivered in a manner similar to that of conventional coal-burning power plants.

Palmer understood the concept of fission only in the sense that it was similar to cell division in biology. The energy was produced in the splitting: that was the value and the magic of nuclear fuel.

Outside, the twin cooling towers gave off steam like giant beakers of concrete.

Palmer marveled. Here was the final piece of the puzzle. The last tumbler falling into place.

This was the moment of the bolt sliding free, just before the great vault door is opened.

As he watched steam clouds drift off into the ominous sky like ghosts rising from great boiling cauldrons, he remembered Chernobyl. The black village of Pripyat, where he had first encountered the Master. The reactor accident was, like the concentration camps in World War II, a lesson for the Master. The human race had shown the Master the way. They had provided the very tools for their own demise.

All of it underwritten by Eldritch Palmer.

He's been out there turning folks for free.

Ah, Dr. Goodweather. But the first shall be last, and the last shall be first. That was how it was supposed to work, according to the Bible.

But this wasn't the Bible. This was America.

The first should be first.

At once, Palmer knew how his business partners felt after dealing with him. Like they'd been punched in the gut with the same hand they just shook.

You think you're working with somebody, until you realize: you're working *for* them.

Why make you wait in line?

Indeed.

Zack pulled away from Nora's hand when his iPod fell to the tunnel floor. It was stupid, it was a reflex, but his mom had bought it for him, even paying for tunes she didn't care for very much, and sometimes hated. When he held the magical little device in his hand and lost himself in the music, he was losing himself in her as well.

"Zachary!"

Weird for Nora to use his full name, but it worked, straightening him up fast. She looked frantic, holding on to her mother near the front of the train. Zack felt something extra for Nora now, something they had in common, seeing her mother so sick: both of their mothers were lost to them, and yet still partly there.

Zack grabbed the music player and shoved it into his jeans pocket, leaving his tangled earphones behind. The derailed train rocked faintly with howling violence and Nora tried to block it from his view. But he knew. He had seen the windows running red. He had seen the faces. He was half in shock, moving through a terrible dream.

Nora had stopped, staring in horror at something behind him.

Out of the tunnel darkness came small figures moving at great speed. With inhuman agility, these recent human children, none of them older than their early teens, sprang toward them along the tracks.

They were led by a phalanx of blind vampire children, eyes black and burned out. The blind ones moved more strangely, the sighted children overtaking them once they reached the train, emitting horrible little squeals of inhuman joy.

They immediately set upon the passengers fleeing the carnage on the train. Others raced up the tunnel walls and swarmed over the roof of the train like baby spiders crawling out of an egg sac.

And among them—one adult figure moved with evil purpose. A feminine form, shadowed by the dim tunnel light, seemingly directing the onslaught. A possessed mother leading an army of demon children.

A hand gripped the hood of his jacket—it was

Nora—yanking Zack away. He stumbled, turning to run with her, taking Nora's mother's arm under his shoulder and half-dragging the old woman from the train wreck flooding over with mad vampire children.

Nora's indigo light barely illuminated their path along the tracks, brightening the kaleidoscope of colorful and sickly psychedelic vampire excrement. No other passengers followed them.

"Look!" Zack said.

His young eyes spotted a pair of steps leading to a door in the left-hand wall. Nora steered them that way, running up to try the handle. It was stuck, or locked, so she stepped back and kicked at it with the heel of her shoe again and again until the handle came down and the door popped open.

Through the other side was an identical platform and two steps leading down into another tunnel. More train tracks, this the southern tube of the tunnel, heading eastbound from New Jersey to Manhattan.

Nora slammed the door, shutting it as hard as she could, then hustled them down onto the tracks.

"Hurry," she said. "Keep moving. We can't fight them all."

They pushed farther into the dark tunnel. Zack helped Nora, supporting her mother, but it was clear they could not walk like this forever.

They never heard anything behind them—never heard the door bang open—and still they moved as though the vampires were right on their heels. Every second felt like borrowed time.

Nora's mother had lost both her shoes, her nylons torn, her feet cut and bleeding. She said over and over, her voice rising, "I need to rest. I want to go home."

Finally, it was too much. Nora slowed, Zack slowing with her. Nora clamped her hand over her mother's mouth, needing to silence her.

Zack saw Nora's face by the purple light of her lamp. He read the stricken expression on her face as she struggled to carry and silence her mother at the same time.

He realized then that she had to make a terrible decision.

Her mother was trying to peel Nora's hand off her mouth. Nora shrugged down her duffel bag. "Open this," she told him. "I want you to take a knife."

"I already have one." Zack dug into his pocket, pulling out the brown bone handle, unfolding the four-inch silver blade.

"Where did you get that?"

"Professor Setrakian gave it to me."

"Good. Zack. Please listen. Do you trust me?"

Such a strange question. "Yes," he said.

"Listen to me. I need you to hide. To get down and crawl underneath this overhang." The track sides were buttressed about two feet from the ground, the angle beneath them cloaked in shadow. "Lie down under there and hold that knife close to your chest. Stay in the shadow. I know it's dangerous. I won't be . . . I won't be long, I promise. Anyone comes by and stops near you, anyone who isn't me—*anyone*—you cut them with that. Do you understand?"

"I . . ." He had seen the faces of the passengers on the train, pressed against the windows. "I understand."

"The throat, the neck—anywhere you can. Keep cutting and stabbing until they fall. Then run ahead and hide again. Understand?"

He nodded, tears rolling down his cheeks.

"Promise me."

Zack nodded again.

"I will be right back. If I am gone too long, you will know it. And then I want you to start running." She pointed toward New Jersey. "That way. All the way. Stopping for nothing. Not even me. All right?"

"What are you going to do?"

But Zack knew. He was certain he knew. And so was Nora.

Nora's mother was biting her hand, forcing Nora to remove it from her mouth. She gripped him in a half-hug, mashing his face into her side. He felt her kiss the crown of his head. Then her mother resumed yelling, and Nora had to cover her mouth again. "Be brave," she told him. "Go."

Zack got down onto his back and wriggled in underneath the overhang, not even thinking about the usual things like rats or mice. He gripped the bone handle tightly, holding the knife to his chest like a crucifix, and listened as Nora struggled to lead her mother away.

* * *

Fet sat in the idling DPW van, waiting. He wore a reflector vest over his usual coveralls, and a hard hat. He was going over the sewer map by the dashboard light.

The old man's makeshift silver chemical weapons were in back, buffeted with rolled towels to prevent them from sliding around. He was worried about this plan. Too many moving parts. He checked the rear door of his shop, waiting for the old man to appear.

Inside, Setrakian adjusted the collar on his cleanest shirt, his gnarled fingers tightening the loops of his bow tie. He pulled out one of his small, silver-backed mirrors in order to check the fit. He was dressed in his best suit.

He put down the mirror and did one last check. His pills! He found the tin and shook the contents gently for luck, cursing himself for almost forgetting it, sliding it inside his jacket pocket. There. Done.

On his way to the door, he looked one last time at the specimen jar that held the remains of his wife's vivisected heart. He had irradiated it with black light, finally killing the blood worm once and for all. The organ, so long in the grip of the parasitic virus, was now blackening with decay.

Setrakian looked upon it as one's gaze falls upon a beloved's gravestone. He meant it to be the last thing he saw of this place. For he was certain he was never coming back.

* * *

Eph sat alone on a long, wooden bench against the wall of the squad room.

The FBI agent's name was Lesh, and his chair and desk were set about three feet beyond Eph's reach. Eph's left wrist was manacled to a low steel rail running along the wall just above the bench, like the safety rails in handicapped bathrooms. Eph had to slouch a bit as he sat, keeping his right leg straight out in order to accommodate the knife still hidden in his waistband. No one had frisked him upon his return from Palmer's.

Agent Lesh had a facial tic, an occasional winking of his left eye that made his cheek dance but did not impair his speech. Pictures of school-age children stood in inexpensive frames upon his cubicle desk.

"So," said the agent. "This thing. I don't get it. Is it a virus, or is it a parasite?"

"It's both," said Eph, trying to be reasonable, still hoping to somehow talk his way free. "The virus is delivered by a parasite, in the form of a blood worm. This parasite is exchanged upon infection, through the throat stinger."

Agent Lesh winked involuntarily and scribbled this down on his pad.

So the FBI was starting to figure things out finally—only much too late. Good cops like Agent Lesh operated at the broad bottom end of the pyramid, having no idea that things had long since been decided by those at the very top.

Eph said, "Where are those other two agents?"

"Who's this?"

"The ones who took me into the city on the helicopter."

Agent Lesh stood, getting a better view over the squad-room cubicles. A few dedicated agents remained at work. "Hey, anybody here take Dr. Goodweather up on a bird into the city?"

Grunts and denials. Eph realized he hadn't seen the two men since his return. "I'd say they're gone for good."

"Can't be," said Agent Lesh. "Our orders are to stand by here until further notice."

That didn't sound good at all. Eph looked again at the pictures on Lesh's desk. "You get your family out of the city?"

"We don't live in the city. Too expensive. I drive in from Jersey every day. But yeah, they're out. School got canceled, so my wife took them up to a friend's on Kinnelon Lake."

Not far enough, thought Eph. "Mine are out, too," he said. He leaned forward, as far as his handcuffs—and the table knife against his hip— would allow. "Look, Agent Lesh," said Eph, trying to take him into his confidence. "All this that's happening . . . I know it seems like chaos, like absolute disorder? It's not. Okay? It is not. This is a carefully planned, coordinated attack. And today . . . today it is all coming to a head. I still don't know exactly how, or what. But it is today. And we—you and me both—need to get out of here."

Agent Lesh winked twice. "You're under arrest, doctor. You shot at a man in broad daylight with dozens of witnesses around you, and you would be on your way to a federal arraignment if things weren't so crazy right now and most government offices weren't closed. So you're not going anywhere, and because of you, neither am I. Now— what can you tell me about these?"

Agent Lesh showed him some printouts. Photographs of markings etched on buildings featuring the six-legged, bug-like graffiti rendering.

"Boston," Agent Lesh said. He shuffled them from the front of the pile to the back. "This one from Pittsburgh. Outside Cleveland. Atlanta. Portland, Oregon, three thousand miles away."

Eph said, "I don't know for sure, but I think it's some sort of code. They don't communicate through speech. They need a system of language. They're marking territory, marking progress . . . something like that."

"And this bug design?"

"I know. It's almost like . . . have you heard of automatic writing? The subconscious mind? See, they are all connected on a psychic level. I don't understand it—only that it exists. And like any great intelligence, I think there's a subconscious segment, with this stuff spilling out . . . almost artistically. Expressing itself. You're seeing the same basic designs scrawled on buildings all across the country. It's probably halfway around the world by now."

Agent Lesh dropped the images back onto his desk. He grabbed the back of his neck, massaging it. "And silver, you say? Ultraviolet light? The sun?"

"Check the gun I had. It's here somewhere,

right? Check the bullets. Pure silver. Not because Palmer is a vampire. He's not—not yet. But it was given to me . . ."

"Yeah? Go on? By whom? I'd like to know how it is you know all these things—"

The lights went out. The heat vents went silent, and everyone in the squad room groaned.

"Not again," said Agent Lesh, getting to his feet.

Emergency lights flickered on, the EXIT signs over the doors and every fifth or sixth ceiling panel light all coming on at half- or a quarter-power.

"Beautiful," said Agent Lesh, pulling a flashlight down off a hook on the top of his cubicle partition.

Then the fire alarm went off, whooping through overhead speakers.

"Ah!" shouted Agent Lesh. "Better and better!"

Eph heard a scream from somewhere in the building.

"Hey," yelled Eph. He tugged on the handcuff bar. "Uncuff me. They're coming for us."

"Huh?" Agent Lesh remained where he was, listening for more screams. "Coming for us?"

A crash, and a noise like a door breaking.

"For me!" said Eph. "My gun. You have to get it!"

Agent Lesh focused on listening. He went ahead and unsnapped his own holster.

"No! That won't work! The silver in my gun! Don't you understand? Go get it—!"

Gunshots. Just one floor beneath them.

"Shit!" Agent Lesh started away, drawing his sidearm.

Eph swore and turned his attention to the bar and his handcuffs. He yanked on the rail with both hands—no give whatsoever. He slid the handcuff down first to one end, then the other, hoping to exploit some weak spot, but the bolts were thick, the bar set deeply into the wall. He kicked at it, but couldn't get through.

Eph heard a scream—closer now—and more gunshots. He tried to stand, only able to get three-quarters of the way erect. He tried to pull the wall down.

Shots in the room now. The cubicle walls blocked his view. All he had to go on was the flashes of flame from the agents' weapons—and the agents' screaming.

Eph dug into his pants for the silver table knife. It felt a lot smaller in his hand here than it had inside Palmer's penthouse. He jammed the dull edge in behind the bench at an angle and pulled back on it, hard and fast. The tip snapped off, producing a short but sharp blade like a jailhouse shiv.

A thing came vaulting onto the top of the cubicle wall. It crouched there, balanced on all four limbs. It appeared small in the dim lighting of the squad room, turning its head in a weird, searching manner, scanning without sight, sniffing without a sense of smell.

Its face turned toward Eph, and he knew it was locked in.

It came off the top of the partition walls with

feline agility, and Eph saw that the child vampire's eyes were blackened like the hot end of a burned-out lightbulb. Its face was turned slightly away from him, its unseeing eyes not trained on his body—and yet somehow it saw him, of that he was certain.

Its physicality was terrifying to Eph, like facing a jaguar in a cage—and being chained to the cage. Eph stood sideways, in the vain hope of protecting his throat, his silver blade out toward the feeler, who sensed the weapon. Eph moved laterally as the handcuff rail would allow, the creature tracking him to the left, and then back toward the right, its head snakelike upon its swollen neck.

Then it struck, its stinger whipping out, shorter than an adult vampire's, Eph just reacting in time to swipe at it with his blade. Whether he cut it or not, he had made impact, fending off the approach, the feeler skittering backward like a kicked dog.

"GET OUTTA HERE!" yelled Eph, trying to command it as he would an animal, but the feeler only looked at him with its unseeing eyes. When two more vampires—regular monsters, red human blood staining their shirtfronts—turned the corner around the partitions, Eph understood that the feeler had summoned backup.

Eph waved his little silver knife, making like a madman. Trying to scare them more than they were scaring him.

It didn't work.

The creatures split up, pouncing from both

sides, Eph slashing at one's arm, then the other's. The silver hurt them, enough to open their limbs and let some whiteness flow.

Then one gripped his knife arm. The other got him by his opposite shoulder, holding his head by the hair.

They didn't take him right away. They were waiting for the feeler. Eph struggled as much as he could, but he was overmatched and chained to the wall. The fever heat of these atrocities, and the stench of their deadness, nauseated him. He tried to throw his knife, flipping the blade at one of them, but it simply slipped from his grip.

The feeler came up on him slowly, a predator savoring its kill. Eph fought to keep his chin down, but the hand in his hair hauled his head back, exposing his throat to the small creature.

Eph howled in defiance in his last moment— when the back part of the feeler's head exploded into a white mist. Its body dropped straight down, twitching, and Eph felt the vampires on either side of him release their grip.

Eph shoved one away, kicking the other off the bench.

Humans rounded the corner then, a couple of Latinos armed to the teeth with tools to fuck up a vampire's night. One vamp got the silver skewer as he tried to scramble up and over the partitions, away from a UVC lamp. The other made a stand, trying to fight—receiving a kick to the knee that dropped him, followed by a silver bolt into his skull.

Then came a third guy, a hulking Mexican

man, probably in his sixties but, old as he appeared, the behemoth was incredibly effective at dispatching vampires left and right.

Eph pulled his legs up onto the bench in order to avoid the spray of white blood on the floor, the worms looking for a new body to host them.

The leader stepped forward, a Mexican kid, leather-gloved, bright-eyed, a bandolier of silver bolts crisscrossing his chest. His black boots, Eph saw, were fronted with toe-plates of white-spattered silver.

"You Dr. Goodweather?" he said.

Eph nodded.

"My name is Augustin Elizalde," the kid said. "The pawnbroker sent us to get you."

Alongside Fet, Setrakian entered the lobby of Sotheby's headquarters at 77th Street and York, asking to be shown to the registration room. He presented a bank check, drawn on a Swiss account, which, after a landline telephone call, cleared instantly.

"Welcome to Sotheby's, Mr. Setrakian."

He was assigned paddle #23 and an attendant showed him to the elevator to the tenth floor. They stopped him outside the door to the auction floor, asking that he check his coat and his wolf-handled staff. Setrakian did so reluctantly, accepting a plastic ticket in return and slipping it inside the watch pocket of his vest. Fet was admitted inside the auction gallery, but only those with paddles were allowed into the seated bidding area. Fet remained behind, standing in back with a view of the entire room, thinking it was perhaps better this way.

The auction was held under intense security. Setrakian took a seat in the fourth row. Not too close, not far away either. He sat on the aisle with his numbered paddle resting on his leg. The stage in front of him was lit, a white-gloved steward pouring water into a glass for the auctioneer, then disappearing into a concealed service entrance. The viewing area was stage left, a brass easel awaiting the first few catalog items. An overhead video screen showed the Sotheby's name.

The first ten or fifteen rows were nearly full, with intermittent empty chairs in back. And yet some of the participants were clearly seat-fillers, employees hired to fill out the bidding audience, their eyes lacking the steely attentiveness of a true buyer. Both sides of the room between the row ends and the moveable walls—set far back for maximum occupancy—were packed, as was the rear. Many of the spectators wore masks and gloves.

An auction is as much theater as marketplace, and the entire affair had a distinctly fin-de-siècle feel: a final burst of flamboyant spending, a last-gasp display of capitalism in the face of over-whelming economic doom. Most of the attendees were gathered simply for the show. Like well-dressed mourners at a funeral service.

Excitement mounted as the auctioneer ap-peared. Anticipation rippled throughout the room while he ran through his opening remarks and the ground rules for bidders. And then he gaveled the auction underway.

The first few items were minor baroque paintings, hors d'oeuvres to whet the bidders' appetites for the main course.

Why did Setrakian feel so tense? So out of sorts, so paranoid suddenly? The deep pockets of the Ancients were today his deep pockets. It was inevitable that the long-sought book would soon be in his hands.

He felt strangely exposed, sitting where he was. He felt . . . observed, not passively, but by knowing eyes. Penetrating and familiar.

He located the source of his paranoia behind a pair of smoke-tinted glasses, three rows behind him on the opposite aisle. The eyes belonged to a figure dressed in a suit of dark fabric, wearing black leather gloves.

Thomas Eichhorst.

His face appeared smoothed and stretched, his body overall looking too well-preserved. It was flesh-colored makeup and a wig, certainly . . . yet there was something else besides. Could it have been surgery? Had some mad doctor been retained to keep his appearance close to that of a human, in order that he might walk and mix with the living? Even though they were hidden behind the Nazi's glasses, Setrakian felt a chill knowing that Eichhorst's eyes had connected with his.

Abraham had been merely a teen when he entered the camp—and so it was with young eyes that he looked upon the former commandant of

Treblinka now. He experienced that same spike of fear, combined with an unreasonable panic. This evil being—while he was still a mere human—had dictated life and death inside that death factory. Sixty-four years ago . . . and now the dread came back to Setrakian as though it had been yesterday. This monster, this beast—now multiplied a hundredfold.

Acid burned the old man's throat, nearly choking him.

Eichhorst nodded to Setrakian, ever so gently. Ever so *cordially*. He appeared to smile—but indeed, it was not a smile, just a way of opening his mouth enough to give Setrakian a glimpse of the tip of his stinger inside, flickering at his rouged lips.

Setrakian turned back to face the dais. He hid the trembling of his crooked hands, an old man ashamed at his boyhood fright.

Eichhorst had come for the book. He would battle for it in the place of the Master, bankrolled by Eldritch Palmer.

Setrakian went into his pocket for his pillbox. His arthritic fingers worked clumsily and doubly hard, as he did not wish Eichhorst to see and enjoy his distress.

He slipped the nitroglycerin pill discreetly beneath his tongue and waited for the pill to take effect. He pledged to himself that, even if it took his very last breath, he would beat this Nazi.

Your heart is erratic, Jew.

Setrakian did not react outwardly to the voice

invading his head. He worked hard to ignore this most unwelcome guest.

In his vision, the auctioneer and the stage disappeared, as did all of Manhattan and the continent of North America. Setrakian saw for the moment only the wire fences of the camp. He saw the dirt muddied with blood and the emaciated faces of his fellow craftsmen.

He saw Eichhorst sitting atop his favorite steed. The horse was the only living thing inside the camp to which he showed any hint of affection, by way of carrots and apples—enjoying feeding the beast right in front of starving prisoners. Eichhorst liked to dig his heels into the horse's sides, making him whinny and rear up. Eichhorst also enjoyed practicing his marksmanship with a Ruger while sitting atop the riled horse. At each assembly, a worker was executed at random. Three times it was a man standing directly next to Setrakian.

I noticed your bodyguard when you entered.

Did he mean Fet? Setrakian turned and saw Fet among the onlookers standing in back, near a pair of well-tailored bodyguards flanking the exit. In his exterminator's coveralls, he appeared completely out of place.

Fetorski, is it not? Pureblood Ukrainian is an exceedingly rare vintage. Bitter, salty, but with a strong finish. You should know, I am a connoisseur of human blood, Jew. My nose never lies. I recognized his bouquet when you entered. As well as the line of his jaw. You don't remember?

The beast's words unnerved Setrakian. Because he hated their source, and because they had, to Setrakian's ear, the ring of truth.

In the camp of his mind's eye, he saw a large man wearing the black uniform of the Ukrainian guards, dutifully gripping the bridle of Eichhorst's mount with gloves of black leather, handing the commandant his Ruger.

It cannot be a mistake that you should be here with the descendant of one of your tormentors?

Setrakian closed his eyes on Eichhorst's taunts. He cleared his mind, returning his focus to the task at hand. He thought, in a mind-voice as loud as he could make it, in the hope that the vampire would hear him: *You will be even more surprised to learn who else I am partnered with this day.*

Nora dug out the night-vision monocular and hung it over the Mets ball cap on her head. Closing one eye turned the North River Tunnel green. "Rat vision," Fet liked to call it, but was she ever grateful for this invention at that moment.

The tunnel area was clear ahead of her, into the intermediate distance. But she could find no exit. No hiding place. Nothing.

She was alone now with her mother, having put enough space between them and Zack. Nora tried not to look at her, even with the scope. Her mother was breathing hard, barely able to keep pace. Nora had her by her arm, practically carrying her over the stones between the tracks, feeling the vampires at their back.

Nora realized she was looking for the right place to do this. The best place. This thing she was contemplating was a horror. The voices in her head—no one else's but her own—offered countervailing arguments:

You can't do this.

You cannot hope to save both your mother and Zack. You have to choose.

How can you choose a boy over your mother?

Choose one or lose both.

She had a good life.

Bullshit. We all have good lives, exactly until the moment they end.

She gave you life.

But if you don't do this now, you are giving her over to vampires. Cursing her for all eternity.

Alzheimer's has no cure either. She is getting progressively worse. She has already changed from the woman who was your mother. How is that different from vampirism?

She poses no threat to others.

Only to yourself—and Zack.

You will have to destroy her anyway when she returns for you, her Dear One.

You told Eph he needed to destroy Kelly.

Her dementia is such that she won't even know.

But you will know.

Bottom line: will you also do yourself in before you are turned?

Yes.

But that is *your* choice.

And it is never an either/or. Never clear-cut. It happens too fast; they are upon you, and you are gone. You

*must act in advance of the turning. You have to antici-
pate it.*

And yet there are no guarantees.

*You cannot release someone before they are turned.
You can only tell yourself that this is what you hope you
did. And wonder forever if you were right.*

It is still murder.

*Will you also turn the knife on Zack if the end is im-
minent?*

Maybe. Yes.

You would hesitate.

Zack has a better chance of surviving an attack.

So you would trade the old for the new.

Maybe. Yes.

Nora's mother said to her, "When in the hell is
your lousy father going to get here?"

Nora came back to the moment. She felt too
sick to cry. It was indeed a cruel world.

A howl echoed through the long tunnel, chill-
ing Nora.

She went around behind her mother's back.
She could not look her in the face. She tightened
her grip on her knife, raising it in order to bring
it down into the back of the old woman's neck.

But all of this was nothing.

She didn't have it in her heart, and she knew
this.

Love is our downfall.

Vampires had no guilt. That was their great advantage. They never hesitated.

And, as though to prove this point, Nora
looked up to find herself being stalked along each
side of the tunnel. Two vampires had crept up on

her while she was distracted, their eyes glowing white-green in her monocular.

They did not know that she could see them. They did not understand night-vision technology. They assumed that she was like all the rest of the passengers—lost in the darkness, wandering blind.

"You sit here, Mama," said Nora, nudging her knees out, lowering her to the tracks. Otherwise, she would go wandering off. "Papa's on his way."

Nora turned and walked toward the two vampires, moving directly between them without looking at either one. Peripherally, they left the stone walls in their loose-jointed way.

Nora took a deep breath before the kill.

These vampires became the recipients of her homicidal angst. She lunged first at the one on the left, slashing it faster than the creature could leap. The vampire's bitter cry rang in her ears as she whipped around and faced the other, who was eyeing her sitting mother. The creature turned back toward Nora from its crouch, its mouth open for the stinger strike.

A splash of white filled her scope like the rage flaring in her head. She slaughtered her would-be attacker, chest heaving, eyes stinging with tears.

She looked back the way she came. Had these two passed Zack to get to her? Neither one appeared flush from a meal, though the night vision couldn't give her an accurate read of their pallor.

Nora grabbed her lamp and turned it on the corpses, frying the blood worms before they had a chance to wriggle over the rocks toward her mother. She irradiated her own knife as well, then switched off the lamp, returning to help her mother to her feet.

"Is your father here?" she said.

"Soon, Mama," said Nora, hurrying her back toward Zack, tears running down her cheeks. "Soon."

Setrakian didn't bother getting in on the bidding for the *Occido Lumen* until the price crossed the $10 million threshold. The rapid pace of the bidding was fueled not only by the extraordinary rarity of the item but also by the circumstances of the auction—this sense that the city was going to come crumbling down at any moment, that the world was changing forever.

At $15 million, the bidding increments rose to $300,000.

At $20 million, $500,000.

Setrakian did not have to turn around to know whom he was bidding against. Others, attracted by the "cursed" nature of the book, jumped in early but fell away once the pace reached an eight-figure frenzy.

The auctioneer called for a brief break in the action at $25 million, reaching for his water glass—but really only stoking the drama. He took a moment to remind those present of the highest auction price ever paid for a book: $30.8 million for da Vinci's Codex Leicester in 1994.

Setrakian now felt the eyes of the room upon him. He kept his attention focused on the *Lumen*, the heavy, silver-covered book brilliantly displayed under glass. It lay open, its facing pages projected upon two large video screens. One was filled with handwritten text, the other showcasing an image of a silver-colored human figure with broad white wings, standing in witness of a distant city being destroyed by a storm of yellow and red flame.

The bidding resumed, rising quickly. Setrakian fell back into a rhythm of raising and lowering his paddle.

The next genuine audience gasp came as they crossed the $30 million threshold.

The auctioneer pointed across the aisle from Setrakian for $30.5 million. Setrakian countered up at $31 million. It was the most expensive book purchase in history now—but what did such landmarks matter to Setrakian? To mankind?

The auctioneer called for $31.5 million, and got it.

Setrakian countered with $32 million before even being prompted.

The auctioneer looked back to Eichhorst, but then, before he had a chance to request the next bid, an attendant appeared, interrupting him. The auctioneer, showing just the right amount of pique, stepped away from the podium to confer with her.

He stiffened at the news, ducked his head, then nodded.

Setrakian wondered what was happening.

The steward then came around off the dais, and began walking up the aisle toward him. Setrakian watched her approach in confusion—then watched as she passed him, going three more rows back, stopping before Eichhorst.

She knelt in the aisle, whispering something to him.

"You may speak to me right here," said Eichhorst—his lips moving in a pantomime of human speech.

The steward spoke further, attempting to preserve the bidder's privacy as best she could.

"That is ridiculous. There is some mistake."

The steward apologized, but remained firm.

"Impossible." Eichhorst rose to his feet. "You will suspend the auction while I rectify this situation."

The steward glanced quickly back at the auctioneer, and then up at the Sotheby's officials watching from behind balcony glass high along the walls, like guests observing a surgery.

The steward turned to Eichhorst and said, "I am afraid, sir, that is just not possible."

"I must insist."

"Sir . . ."

Eichhorst turned to the auctioneer, pointing at him with his paddle. "You will hold your gavel until I am allowed to make contact with my benefactor."

The auctioneer returned to his microphone. "The rules of auction are quite clear on this point, sir. I am afraid that without a viable line of credit—"

"I indeed do have a viable line of credit."

"Sir, our information is that it has just been

rescinded. I am very sorry. You will have to take up the matter with your bank—"

"My bank! On the contrary, we will complete the bidding here and now, and then I will straighten out this irregularity!"

"I am sorry, sir. The house rules are the same as they have been for decades, and cannot be altered, not for anyone." The auctioneer looked out over the audience, resuming the bidding. "I have $32 million."

Eichhorst raised his paddle. "$35 million!"

"Sir, I am sorry. The bid is $32 million. Do I hear $32.5?"

Setrakian sat with his paddle on his leg, ready. "$32.5?"

Nothing.

"$32 million, going once."

"$40 million!" said Eichhorst, standing in the aisle now.

"$32 million, going twice."

"I object! This auction must be canceled. I must be allowed more time—"

"$32 million. Lot 1007 is sold to bidder #23. Congratulations."

The gavel came down to ratify the sale; the room burst into applause. Hands reached toward Setrakian in congratulations, but the old man got to his feet as quickly as possible and walked to the front of the room, where he was met by another steward.

"I would like to take possession of the book immediately," he informed her.

"But, sir, we have some paperwork—"

"You may clear the payment, including the house's commission, but I am taking possession of the book, and I am doing so now."

Gus's battered Hummer wove and bashed its way back across the Queensboro Bridge. As they returned to Manhattan, Eph spotted dozens of military vehicles staged at 59th Street and Second Avenue, in front of the entrance to the Roosevelt Island Tramway. The larger, canopied trucks read FORT DRUM in black stencil, and two white buses, as well as some Jeeps, read USMA WEST POINT.

"Shutting down the bridge?" said Gus, his gloved hands tight upon the steering wheel.

"Maybe enforcing the quarantine," said Eph.

"You think they are with us or against us?"

Eph saw personnel in combat fatigues pulling a tarp down off a large, truck-mounted machine gun—and he felt his heart lift a little. "I'm going to say with us."

"I hope so," said Gus, swinging hard toward uptown. "Because if not, this is gonna get even more fucking interesting."

They arrived at 72nd and York just as the street battle was getting underway. Vamps came streaming out of the brick-tower nursing home across the street from Sotheby's—the aged residents imbued with new motility and *strigoi* strength.

Gus killed the engine and popped the trunk. Eph, Angel, and the two Sapphires jumped out and started grabbing silver.

"I guess he won it after all," said Gus, ripping open a carton, handing Eph two vases of painted glass with narrow necks, gasoline sloshing inside.

"Won what?" said Eph.

Gus wicked a rag into each and then flicked open a silver-plated Zippo, igniting them. He took one vase from Eph and walked out into the street away from the Hummer. "Put your shoulder into it, homes," said Gus. "On three. One. Two. *Yahh!*"

They catapulted the economy-sized Molotov cocktails over the heads of the marauding vampires. The vases shattered, igniting immediately, liquid flame opening up and spreading instantly like twin pools of hell. Two Carmelite sisters went up first, their brown-and-white habits taking to the flame like sheets of newspaper. Then went the multitude of vampires in bathrobes and housecoats, squealing. The Sapphires came on next, skewering the engulfed creatures, finishing them off—only to see more come charging down 71st Street, like maniac firefighters answering a psychic five-alarm call.

A couple of burning vampires charged on, flames trailing, and only stopped a foot or so away from Gus after being riddled with silver bullets.

"Where the hell are they already?" yelled Gus, looking to Sotheby's entrance. The tall, thin sidewalk trees out front burned like hellish sentries outside the auction house.

Eph saw building guards rushing to lock the revolving doors inside the glass lobby. "Come on!" he yelled, and they fought their way past the burning trees. Gus wasted some silver bolts on the doors, puncturing and weakening the glass before Angel charged through.

Setrakian leaned heavily on his oversize walking stick in the elevator going down. The auction had drained him, and yet there was so much more to do. Fet stood at his side, his weapon pack on his back, the $32 million book in bubble wrap under his arm.

To Setrakian's right, one of the auction house's security guards waited with hands clasped over his belt buckle.

Chamber music played over the panel speaker. A string quartet, Dvořák.

"Congratulations, sir," said the security guard, to break the silence.

"Yes," said Setrakian. He noticed the white wire in the man's brown ear. "Does your radio work in this elevator, by any chance?"

"No, sir, it does not."

The elevator stopped abruptly, all three men grabbing for the wall to steady themselves. The car started down again at once, then again stopped. The number on the overhead display read 4.

The guard pressed the DOWN button, then the 4 button, thumbing each one numerous times.

While the guard was so engaged, Fet drew a sword from his pack and faced the elevator door. Setrakian twisted the grip of his walking stick, exposing the silver shaft of his hidden blade.

The first bang against the door shook the guard, making him jump back.

The second blow produced a serving bowl–size dent.

The guard reached out his hand to feel the convexity. He began to say, "What the—"

The door slid open, and pale hands reached inside, pulling him out.

Fet barreled out after him with the book clutched under his arm, lowering his shoulder and driving forward like a running back taking the pigskin through an entire defensive line. He plowed the vampires straight back against the wall, Setrakian exiting behind him, his silver sword flashing, killing a path toward the main floor.

Fet slashed and chopped, fighting at close quarters with the creatures, feeling their inhuman warmth, their acidic white blood spurting onto his coat. He reached for the security guard with the fingers of his sword hand, but found he could do nothing for him, the guard disappearing to the floor beneath a huddle of hungry vampires.

With wide, sweeping slices, Setrakian cleared the way to the front railing overlooking the interior four-story drop. Outside, he saw bodies burning in the street, trees on fire, a melee at the building entrance. Inside, looking straight down, he saw the gangbanger Gus alongside his older Mexican friend. It was the limping ex-wrestler who looked up, pointing out Setrakian.

"Here!" Setrakian called back to Fet. Fet extricated himself from the pile-up, checking his clothes for blood worms as he came running. Setrakian pointed out the wrestler.

"You sure?" said Fet.

Setrakian nodded, and Fet, with a great scowl, held the *Occido Lumen* out over the railing, giving the wrestler a moment to limp over beneath him. Gus slashed a demon in the wrestler's way, and Setrakian saw someone else—yes, it was Ephraim—warding others away with a lamp of ultraviolet light.

Fet released the precious book, watching it slowly turn as it fell.

Four stories below them, Angel caught it in his arms like a baby thrown from a burning building.

Fet turned, now able to fight two-handedly, sliding a dagger from the bottom of his pack and leading Setrakian to the escalators. The motorized staircases ran crisscross, side-by-side. Vampires on their way up—summoned to battle by the will of the Master—jumped tracks where the stairways crossed. Fet dispatched them with the tread of his boot and the tip of his sword, sending them sprawling down the moving stairs.

On the bottom flight, Setrakian looked back up through the gap. He saw Eichhorst high above on one of the upper floors, looking down.

The others had done most of the work for them in the lobby. Released vampire corpses lay twisted on the floor, faces and clawed hands frozen in a tableau of white-splattered agony. More vampire drones were pounding on the glass entrance, with still others on the way.

Gus led them back out through the smashed doors onto the sidewalk. Vampires came swarming from 71st and 72nd to the west, and York Avenue north and south. They came up out of the streets, rising through displaced manholes in the intersections. Fighting them off was like trying to bail out of a sinking ship, two vampires arriving for every one destroyed.

A pair of black Hummers rounded the corner hard, headlights angry, front grilles bumping down vampires, rugged tires squashing their bodies. A team of hunters stepped out, hooded and armed with crossbows, and immediately made their presence known. Vampire killing vampire, the drones getting mowed down by the elite guard.

Setrakian knew they had arrived either to escort him and the book directly to the Ancients, or to take possession of the Silver Codex outright. Neither option suited him. He remained close to the wrestler, who carried the book under his arm; his lumbering pace suited Setrakian's slow legs. Upon learning the wrestler's moniker, "The Silver Angel," Setrakian had to smile.

Fet led the way to the corner of 72nd and York. The manhole he wanted had already been popped open, and he grabbed Creem and sent him down first, to clear the hole of vampires. He let Angel and Setrakian down next, the wrestler barely fitting inside the hole. Then Eph, without any questions, climbing right down the iron ladder rungs. Gus and the rest of the Sapphires hung back in order to allow the vampires to close in on them, then went down themselves, Fet disappearing below just as the ring of mayhem collapsed on him.

"Other way!" he yelled down to them. "Other way!"

They had started west along the sewer tunnel, toward the heart of the island underground, but Fet dropped down and led them east, underneath one long block that dead-ended over FDR Drive. The trough of the tunnel carried a measly trickle of water; lack of human activity in surface Manhattan meant fewer showers, fewer flushes.

"All the way to the end!" said Fet, his voice booming inside the stone tube.

Eph came up alongside Setrakian. The old man was slowing, the nub of his walking stick splashing in the water stream. "Can you make it?" said Eph.

"Have to," said Setrakian.

"I saw Palmer. Today is the day. The last day."

Setrakian said, "I know it."

Eph patted Angel's arm, the one that held the bubble-wrapped book. "Here." Eph took the bundle from him, and the hobbling Mexican giant took Setrakian's arm, helping the old man along.

Eph looked at the wrestler as they rushed, filled with questions he knew not how to ask.

"Here they come!" said Fet.

Eph looked back. Mere shapes in the dark tunnel, to his eyes, coming at them like a dark rush of drowning water.

Two of the Sapphires turned back to fight. "No!" cried Fet. "Don't bother! Just get through here!"

Fet slowed between two long wooden cases

strapped to pipes along the tunnel walls. They looked like speaker bars, set vertically, angled in toward the tunnel. To each, he had rigged a simple switch wire, both of which he gathered in his hands now.

"Down the side!" he yelled to the others behind him. "Through the panel."

But none of them turned the corner. The sight of the onrushing vampires and Fet standing alone in the tunnel holding the triggers to Setrakian's contraption was too compelling.

Out of the darkness came the first faces, red-eyed, mouths open. Tumbling over one another in an all-out race to be the first to attack the humans, *strigoi* surged toward them without any regard for their fellow vampires or themselves. A stampede of sickness and depravity, the fury of the overturned hive.

Fet waited, and waited, and waited, until they were nearly upon him. His voice rose in a yell that started in his throat, but by the end seemed to come straight from his mind, a howl of human perseverance into the gale force of a hurricane.

Their hands reached out, the tide of vampires about to overwhelm him—as he flicked both switches.

The effect was something like the ignition of a giant camera flashbulb. The twin devices went off simultaneously in a single explosion of silver. An expulsion of chemical matter that eviscerated the vampires in a wave of devastation. Those in the rear went as quickly as those at the vanguard, because there was no shadow to hide in, the silver particulate burning through them like radiation, smashing their viral DNA.

The silver tinge lingered in the moments after the great purge, like a shiny snowfall, Fet's howl fading into the emptied tunnel as the shredded matter that was the once-human vampires settled to the tunnel floor.

Gone. As though he had teleported them somewhere else. Like taking a picture, only once the flash faded, no one was there.

No one complete, at least.

Fet released the triggers and turned back at Setrakian.

Setrakian said, "Indeed."

They followed another ladder, leading down to a walkway with a railing. At the end was a door that opened onto an under-sidewalk grate, the surface visible above them. Fet climbed up the boxes he had set as steps, and popped the loosened grate free with his shoulder.

They emerged at the 73rd Street ramp entrance onto FDR Drive. A few strays blundered into them as they rushed across the six-lane parkway over the dividing concrete barriers, moving around abandoned cars toward the East River.

Eph looked back, seeing vampires dropping down off the high balcony that was the courtyard at the end of 72nd Street. They came swarming out of 73rd along the parkway. Eph worried that they were backing themselves up against the river, with blood-hungry revenants closing on all sides.

But on the other side of a low iron fence was a

landing, a municipal dock of sorts, though it was too dark for Eph to see what it was for. Fet went over first, moving with surly confidence, and so Eph followed with all the others.

Fet ran to the end of the landing, and Eph saw it now: a tugboat, large tires tied all the way around its sides, acting as fenders. They climbed onto the main deck, Fet running up into the wheelhouse. The engine started with a cough and a roar, and Eph untied the aft end. The boat lurched at first, Fet pushing it too hard, then launched away from the island.

Out on the West Channel, floating a few dozen yards off the edge of Manhattan, Eph watched the horde of vampires clamor to the edge of FDR Drive. They bunched there, trailing the boat along its slow southern path, unable to venture out over moving water.

The river was a safe zone. A no-vamp's-land.

Beyond the plunderers, Eph looked up at the looming buildings of the darkened city. Behind him, above Roosevelt Island, in the middle of the East River, were pockets of daylight—not pure sunlight, for it was evidently an overcast day, but clarity—between the smoke-veiled landmasses of Manhattan and Queens.

They approached the Queensboro Bridge, gliding underneath the high cantilever span. A bright flash streaked across the Manhattan skyline, turning Eph's head. Then another went up, like a modest firework. Then a third.

Illumination flares, in orange and white.

A vehicle came tearing up FDR Drive toward

the throng of vampires following the boat. It was a Jeep, soldiers in camouflage standing out of the back, firing automatic weapons into the crowd.

"The Army!" said Eph. He felt something he hadn't felt in some time: hope. He looked around for Setrakian, and, not seeing him, headed into the main cabin.

Nora finally found a door, leading not to any sort of exit from the tunnel but into a deep storage closet. There was no lock—the planners never anticipated pedestrians one hundred feet below the Hudson—and inside she found safety equipment, such as replacement bulbs for signal lights, orange flags and vests, and an old cardboard box of flares. Flashlights also, but the batteries were all corroded.

She evened out a pile of sandbags in the corner to fashion a seat for her mother, then grabbed a handful of flares, throwing them into her bag.

"Mama. Please, please, be quiet. Stay here. I am coming back. I am."

Nora's mother sat on the cold throne of sandbags with a curious look about the closet. "Where did you put the cookies?"

"All gone, Mama. You sleep now. Rest."

"Here? In the pantry?"

"Please. It's a surprise—for Papa." Nora was backing out through the door. "Don't move until he comes for you."

She closed the door quickly, scanning the tunnel for vampires with her scope, then dumping two sandbags in front of the door to hold it shut. She then went racing back toward Zack, simultaneously leading her own scent away from her mother.

She had taken the coward's way out, she supposed—stuffing her poor mother inside a closet—but at least this way there was hope.

She continued back along the eastbound side of the tunnel, looking for the place where Zack had hidden. Things looked different through the soupy green light of the monocular. Her marker had been a stripe of white paint along the low side of the tunnel—but she could not locate it now. She thought again of those two vampires who had come up on her, and was leaping with anxiety.

"Zack!" A yelled whisper. Foolhardy, but concern trumped reason. She had to be near where she had left him. "Zack—it's Nora! Where are . . . ?"

What she saw before her chased the voice from her throat. Illuminated in her monocular, illustrated on the broad side of the tunnel, was a vast graffiti mural rendered with exceptional technique. It depicted a great, faceless humanlike creature with two arms, two legs, and two magnificent wings.

She realized intuitively that this was the final iteration of the six-petal tags they had been finding all around town. The earlier flowers, or bugs: those were icons, analogs, abstractions. Cartoons of this fearsome being.

The image of this broad-winged creature, and the manner in which it was rendered—at once both naturalistic and extraordinarily evocative—terrified her in a way she could not begin to understand. How eerie was this ambitious work of street art appearing in this dark tunnel so deep beneath the surface of the earth. A brilliant tattoo of extraordinary beauty and menace written upon this bowel of civilization.

An image, she realized at once, intended to be viewed only by vampiric eyes.

A sibilation spun Nora around. In her night-scope, she saw Kelly Goodweather, her face twisted into an expression of want that nearly resembled pain. Her mouth was an open slit, the tip of her stinger flicking like a lizard's tongue, her parted lips bared in a hiss.

Her torn clothes were still soaked from the surface rain, hanging heavily from her thin body, her hair flattened, smears of dirt streaking her flesh. Her eyes, which appeared screaming white in the greenness of Nora's scope, were wide with want.

Nora fumbled out her UVC lamp. She needed to put some hot space between herself and her lover's undead ex-wife—but Kelly came at her with incredible speed, smacking the lamp from her hand before Nora could turn on the switch.

The Luma lamp smashed against the wall and fell to the ground.

Only Nora's silver blade kept Kelly off her, the vampire leaping up and backward onto the low tunnel shelf. She then hurdled over Nora to the other side, Nora tracking her with her long knife. Kelly feigned an attack, then again bounded overhead. This time Nora swiped at her as she passed, dizzied from having to view the agile creature through her scope.

Kelly landed on the other side of the tunnel, a slash of white appearing on the side of her neck. A surface wound only, but enough to get Kelly's attention. The vampire viewed its own white blood on its long hand, then flicked it at Nora, her face turning wicked and fierce.

Nora backed off, reaching into her bag for one of the flares. She heard limbs scrabbling over track stones, and did not need to take her eyes off Kelly to see them.

Three little vampire children, two boys and a girl, summoned by Kelly to assist in taking Nora down.

"Okay," said Nora, twisting the plastic cap off the flare. "You want to do it this way?" She scratched the top of the cap against the red stick and the flare ignited, red flame searing into the darkness. Nora tipped back her scope, able to see with her own eyes now, the flame illuminating their section of the tunnel from ceiling to floor in a nimbus of angry red.

The children loped backward, repelled by the bright light. Nora waved the flare at Kelly, who lowered her chin but did not retreat.

One of the boys came at Nora from the side, emitting a shrill squeal, and Nora stepped into the child with her knife—burying the silver blade deep into its chest, right to the hilt. The child sagged and staggered back—Nora pulling back the blade fast—weakened and dazed.

The child spread its lips, attempting a last-ditch sting—and Nora jammed the hot end of the flare into its mouth.

The creature bucked wildly, Nora hacking at it with her knife, screaming all the while.

The child vampire fell, and Nora pulled out the flare, still lit. She whipped around, anticipating Kelly's rear attack.

But Kelly was gone. Nowhere to be found.

Nora brandished the flare, the two remaining vampire children crouching near their fallen playmate. She made sure that Kelly wasn't on the ceiling or underneath the ledge.

Uncertainty was worse. The children split up, circling around her on either side, and Nora backed up to the wall beneath the giant mural, ready to do battle, determined not to be ambushed.

Eldritch Palmer watched the illumination flares streaking over rooftops uptown. Puny fireworks. Match-strikes in a world of darkness. The helicopter approached him from the north, slowing above. He awaited his visitors on the seventy-eighth floor of the Stoneheart Building.

Eichhorst was first. A vampire wearing a tweed suit was like a pit bull wearing a knit sweater. He held the door open, the Master ducking as it entered, striding, cloaked, across the floor.

Palmer watched all this through the reflection in the windows.

Explain.

The voice sepulchral, edged with fury.

Palmer, having summoned the strength to stand, turned on his weak legs. "I cut off your funding. I closed the line of credit. Simple."

Eichhorst stood to the side, watching with his gloved hands crossed. The Master looked down at Palmer, its raw-red skin inflamed, its eyes crimson and penetrating.

Palmer went on, "It was a demonstration. Of how critical my participation is to your success. It became evident to me that you needed to be reminded of my worth."

They won the book.

This from Eichhorst, whose contempt for Palmer had always been certain, and returned in kind. But Palmer addressed the Master.

"What does it matter at this late moment? Turn me and I will be only too happy to finish off Professor Setrakian myself."

You understand so little. But then, you have never viewed me as anything other than a means to an end. Your end.

"And shouldn't I say the same of you! You, who has withheld your gift from me for so many years. I have given you everything and withheld nothing. Until this moment!"

This book is no mere trophy. It is a chalice of information. It is the last, lingering hope of the pig humans. The final gasp of your race. This, you cannot conceive. Your human perspective is so small.

"Then allow me to see." Palmer stepped toward him, standing only halfway up the Master's cloaked chest. "It is time. Deliver to me what is rightfully mine, and everything you need shall be yours."

The Master said nothing into Palmer's head. He did not move.

But Palmer was fearless. "We have a deal."

Did you stop anything else? Have you disrupted any of the other plans we set in motion?

"None. Everything stands. Now—do we have a deal?"

We do.

The suddenness with which the Master leaned down to him shocked Palmer, made his fragile heart jump. Its face, up close, the blood worms coasting the veins and capillaries just beneath the florid beetroot that was its skin. Palmer's brain released long-forgotten hormones, the moment of conversion upon him. Mentally, he had long ago packed his bags, and yet there was still a burst of trepidation at the first step of the ultimate one-way voyage. He had no quarrel with the improvements the turning would have upon his body; he wondered only what it would do to his long-held consolation and fiercest weapon, his mind.

The Master's hand pressed onto Palmer's bony shoulder like a vulture's talons onto a twig. Its other hand gripped the crown of Palmer's head, turning it to one side, fully extending the old man's neck and throat.

Palmer looked at the ceiling, his eyes losing focus. He heard choir voices in his head. He had never been held by anyone—anything—in their arms like this in his life. He allowed himself to go limp.

He was ready. His breath came in short, excited bursts as the hardened nail of the Master's long, thick middle finger pricked at the flesh sagging over his stretched neck.

The Master saw the sick man's pulse beating through his neck, the man's heart throbbing in anticipation, and the Master felt the call deep within its stinger. He wanted blood.

But it ignored its nature and, with one firm crack, it ripped Eldritch Palmer's head from his torso. It released the head and gripped the spurting body and tore Palmer in half, the body splitting apart easily where the bones of the hips narrowed to the waist. It tossed the bloody pieces of meat to the far wall, where they struck the framed masterworks of human abstract art and fell to the floor.

The Master turned fast, sensing another blood source ticking on the premises. Palmer's manservant, Mr. Fitzwilliam, stood in the doorway. A broad-shouldered human wearing a suit tailored to accommodate weapons of self-defense.

Palmer had wanted this man's body for his turning. He coveted his bodyguard's strength, his physical stature, desiring the man's form for all eternity.

Mr. Fitzwilliam was one of a package with Palmer.

The Master looked into his mind, and showed him this, before flying at him in a blur. Mr. Fitzwilliam first saw the Master all the way across the room, red blood dripping from his enormous hands—and then the Master was bent over him, a stinging, draining sensation like a rod of fire in his throat.

The pain faded after a time. So did Mr. Fitzwilliam's view of the ceiling.

The Master let the man fall where he had drunk him.

Animals.

Eichhorst remained across the wide room, patient as a lawyer.

The Master said:

Let us commence the Night Eternal.

The tugboat drifted down the East River without lights, toward the United Nations. Fet guided the boat along the besieged island, staying only a few hundred yards off the coast. He was no boat captain, but the throttle was easy enough to operate, and, as he had learned in docking the tug at 72nd Street, the thick tire fenders were quite forgiving.

Behind him, at the navigation table, Setrakian sat before the *Occido Lumen*. A single strong lamp made the silver-leaf illustrations glow off the page. Setrakian was absorbed in the work, studying it in a near-trance. He kept a small notebook next to him. A ruled composition school notebook almost half-full with the old man's notes.

The writing in the *Lumen* was densely yet beautifully hand-scribed, as many as one hundred lines to a page. His old, long-ago-broken fingers turned each corner with delicacy and speed.

He analyzed every page, backlighting them,

scanning for watermarks and quickly sketching them as they were discovered. He annotated their exact position and disposition on the page, as these were vital elements in decoding the text laid on them.

Eph stood at his shoulder, alternately looking at the phantasmagoric illustrations and checking the burning island out the wheelhouse window. He noticed a radio near Fet and switched it on, keeping it low so as not to distract Setrakian. It was satellite radio, and Eph searched the news channels until he came across a voice.

A tired female voice, a broadcaster holed up in the Sirius XM headquarters, was operating off some sort of failsafe backup generator. She was working off multiple, fractured sources—Internet, phone, and e-mail—collating reports from around the country and the world, while repeatedly clarifying that she had no way of verifying this information was accurate.

She spoke candidly about vampirism as a virus spreading person-to-person. She detailed a crumbling domestic infrastructure: accidents, some catastrophic, disabling, or otherwise cutting off traffic along key bridges in Connecticut, Florida, Ohio, Washington state, and California. Power outages further isolated certain regions, most prevalent along the coasts. Gas lines in the Midwest. The National Guard and various Army regiments had been ordered into peacekeeping duty in many major metropolitan centers, with reports of military activity in New York and Washington, DC. Fighting had broken out along the border between North and South Korea. Burning mosques in Iraq had triggered rioting, compounded by U.S. peacekeeping efforts there. A series of unexplained explosions in the catacombs beneath Paris had crippled the city. And an eerie series of reports detailed suicide clusters occurring at Victoria Falls in Zimbabwe, Iguazu Falls on the border between Brazil and Argentina, and Niagara Falls in New York.

Eph shook his head at all of this—bewildering, a nightmare, *War of the Worlds* come true—until he heard the report of an Amtrak derailment inside the North River Tunnel, further cutting off the island of Manhattan. The broadcaster moved on to a report of rioting in Mexico City, leaving Eph staring at the radio.

"Derailment," he said.

The radio couldn't answer him.

Fet said, "She didn't say when. Maybe they got through."

Fear spiked in Eph's chest. He felt sick. "They didn't," he said. He knew it. No ESP, no psychic knowledge: he simply knew it. Their escape now struck him as being too good to be true. All his relief, his clear-headedness—gone. A dark pall fell over his mind.

"I have to go there." He turned toward Fet, unable to see anything but the mental image of a derailment and vampire attack. "Bring us in. You have to let me off. I'm going after Zack and Nora."

Fet did not argue, fooling with the steering controls. "Let me find someplace to crash-land."

Eph looked for weapons. Former gang rivals

Gus and Creem were eating junk food out of a convenience-store bag. Gus used his boot to slide their weapon bag toward Eph.

A change in the broadcaster's tone returned their attention to the radio. A nuclear plant accident had been reported on the eastern coast of China. Nothing out of Chinese news agencies, but there were eyewitness accounts of a mushroom cloud visible from Taiwan, as well as seismometer readings near Guangdong indicating an Earth tremor in the neighborhood of a quake registering 6.6 on the Richter scale. The lack of reporting from Hong Kong was said to indicate the possibility of a nuclear electromagnetic pulse, which would turn electrical cables into lightning rods or antennas and have the effect of frying any connected solid-state devices.

Gus said, "Vampires nuking us now? Fuck us." Then he translated for Angel, who was repairing a homemade splint around his knee.

"Madre de Dios," said Angel, crossing himself.

Fet said, "Wait a minute. A nuclear plant accident? That's a meltdown, not a bomb. Maybe a steam explosion on the site—like Chernobyl—but not a detonation. They're designed so that those aren't possible."

"Designed by whom?" Setrakian said this, never looking up from the book.

Fet sputtered. "I don't know—what do you mean?"

"Constructed by whom?"

"Stoneheart," said Eph. "Eldritch Palmer."

"What?" said Fet. "But—nuclear explosions?

Why do that when he's so close to winning the world?"

"There will be more," said Setrakian. His voice came without breath, disembodied, intoned.

Fet said, "What do you mean, more?"

Setrakian said, "Four more. The Ancients were born from the light. The Fallen Light, *Occido Lumen*—and they can only be consumed by it . . ."

Gus got up and went to stand over the old man. The book was open to a two-page spread. A complex mandala in silver, black, and red. On top of it, on tracing paper, Setrakian had laid out the outline of the six-winged angel. Gus said, "It says that?"

Setrakian closed the silver book and got to his feet. "We must return to the Ancients. At once."

Gus said, "Okay," though he was befuddled by this sudden change in course. "To give them the book?"

"No," said Setrakian, finding his pillbox inside his vest pocket, pulling it open with trembling fingers. "The book arrives too late for them."

Gus squinted. "Too late?"

Setrakian struggled to pluck a nitroglycerin pill out of the box. Fet steadied the old man's shaking hand, pinching a nitroglycerin pill and laying it into his wrinkled palm. "You do realize, professor," said Fet, "that Palmer just opened a new nuclear plant on Long Island."

The old man's eyes grew distant and unfocused, as though still dazed by the concentric geometry of the mandala. Then Setrakian placed the pill beneath his tongue and closed his eyes, waiting for its effects to steady his heart.

Zack, after Nora had gone off with her mother, lay in filth beneath the short ledge running the length of the southern tube of the North River Tunnels, hugging the silver blade to his chest. She was coming right back, and he had to listen for her. Not easy over the sound of his wheezing. He realized this only now, and felt around in his pockets, finding his inhaler.

He brought it to his mouth and took two puffs, and felt immediate relief. He thought of the breath in his lungs like a guy trapped inside a net. When Zack got anxious, it was like the guy was fighting the net, pulling at it, winding himself up worse and making everything tight. The puff from Zack's inhaler was like a blast of knockout gas, the guy weakening, going limp, the net relaxing over him.

He put away the inhaler and reaffirmed his grip on the knife. *Give it a name and it's yours forever.* That is what the professor had told him. Zack feverishly raced through his thoughts in search of a name. Trying to focus on anything but the tunnel.

Cars get girl names. Guns get guy names. What do knives get?

He thought of the professor, the man's old, broken fingers, presenting him with the weapon.

Abraham.

That was his first name.

That was the name of the knife.

"Help!"

A man's voice. Someone running through the tunnel—coming nearer. His voice echoing.

"Help me! Anybody there?"

Zack did not move. He didn't even turn his head, only his eyes. He heard the man stumble and fall, and that was when Zack heard the other footsteps. Someone pursuing him. The man got up again, then fell. Or else was thrown down. Zack hadn't realized how close the man was to him. The man kicked and howled out some gibberish like a madman, crawling along one of the rails. Zack saw him then, a form in the darkness, clawing forward while kicking back at his pursuers. He was so near that Zack could feel the man's terror. So near that Zack readied Abraham in his hand, blade pointing out.

One of them landed on the man's back. His yowling was cut short, one of their hands reaching around and entering his open mouth, pulling at his cheek. More hands set upon him—overlarge fingers grabbing at his flesh and his clothes, and dragging him away.

Zack felt the man's madness spread into him. He lay there shivering so hard he thought he was going to give himself away. The man got off another anguished groan, and it was enough to know that they—the children's hands—were pulling him back the other way.

Zack had to run. He had to run off after Nora. He remembered one time playing hide-and-seek in his old neighborhood, and he had burrowed in behind some bushes, listening to the seeker's slow count. He was found last, or almost last, once he realized that one kid was still missing, a younger boy who had joined the game late. And they looked for him a little bit, calling his name, and then lost interest, figuring he had gone back home. But Zack didn't think so. He had seen the glimmer in the young boy's eye when they ran off to hide, the almost-evil anticipation of the hunted wanting to outwit the hunter. Beyond the thrill of the chase: the knowledge of a really clever hiding place.

Clever to a five-year-old's mind. And then Zack knew. He went all the way down the street to the house owned by the old man who yelled at them when kids cut through his backyard. Zack went to the refrigerator lying on its side, still at the bottom of their driveway on the day after trash day. The door had been removed, but now it lay on top of the squash-yellow appliance. Zack pulled it open, breaking the seal, and there was the boy, starting to turn blue. Somehow, with near Hulk-like hide-and-seek strength, the five-year-old had pulled the door of the fridge over him. The boy was fine, except for puking onto the lawn after Zack helped him out, and the old man coming to his door and yelling at them to beat it.

Beat it.

Zack slid out on his back, half-coated in tunnel soot, and started running. He turned on his busted iPod, the cracked screen lighting the floor in front of him in a four-foot nimbus of soft, blue light. He couldn't hear anything, even his own footfalls, so loud was the panic in his head. He assumed he was being chased—could feel hands reaching for the back of his neck—and whether true or not, he ran as though it were.

He wanted to call out Nora's name, but did not, knowing it would give away his position. Abraham's blade scraped the wall of the tunnel, telling him he was veering too far to the right.

Zack saw a burning red flame up ahead. Not a torch, but an angry light, like a flare. It scared him. He was supposed to be running away from trouble, not toward it. He slowed, not wanting to go forward, unable to go back.

He thought about the boy hiding inside the refrigerator. No light, no sound, no air.

The door, dark against the dividing wall, had a sign on it Zack did not bother to read. The handle turned and he went through it, back into the original northbound tunnel. He could smell the smoke the friction of the derailed train caused, along with the noxious stench of ammonia. This was a mistake—he should wait for Nora, she would be looking for him—but on he ran.

Ahead, a figure. At first, he believed that it was Nora. This person also wore a backpack, and Nora had been carrying a bag.

But such optimism was just a trick of his preteen mind.

The hissing sound scared him initially. But Zack saw enough in the faint outer reaches of his light source to tell that this person was involved in an endeavor that did not involve violence. He watched the graceful movements of the person's arm and realized he was spraying paint onto the tunnel wall.

Zack went another step forward. The person was not much taller than he, a sweatshirt hood over his head. There was paint spatter on his elbows and the hem of his black hoodie, his camouflage pants and Converse hi-tops. He was doing up the wall, though Zack could see only a small corner of the mural, which was silver and ruffled in appearance. Under it, the vandal was finishing his tag. PHADE, it read.

All this happened in moments—which was why it did not seem unusual to Zack that someone should have been painting in absolute darkness.

Phade lowered his arm, having finished his signature, then turned toward Zack.

Zack said, "Hey, I don't know what you know, but you gotta get out of this . . ."

Phade slid back the hood covering his face—and it was not a he. Phade was a girl, or had once been a girl, no older than her teens. Phade's face was now inert, unnaturally immobile, like a mask of dead flesh wrapping the malignant biology festering within. Its skin, by Zack's iPod light, had the pallor of pickled flesh, like the color of a fetal pig inside a specimen jar. Zack saw a spill of red down the front of its chin, neck, and sweatshirt. The red stain was not paint.

Zack heard squealing behind him. He turned for a moment—and then whipped around, realizing he had just turned his back on a vampire. As he turned back to Phade, he put out his hand with the knife in it, not knowing that Phade had darted straight at him.

Abraham's blade ran right into Phade's throat. Zack pulled back his hand fast, as though having committed a tragic accident, and white fluid came burbling out of Phade's neck. Phade's eyes rolled wide with a surge of menace, and before Zack knew what he was doing, he had stabbed the vampire four more times in the throat. The can of spray paint *sssss*ed against Phade's leg before falling to the ground.

The vampire collapsed.

Zack stood there with the murder weapon in his hand, holding Abraham like something he had broken and didn't know how to set down.

The patter of advancing vampires woke him up, unseen but bearing down on him out of the darkness. Zack dropped his iPod light, reaching down for the can of silver paint. He got it into his hand and the spray trigger under his finger just as two spiderlike vampire children came screaming out of the dark, stingers flicking in and out of their mouths. The way in which they moved was indescribably wrong, so swift, exploiting the flexibility of youth into dislocated arms and knees, moving impossibly low and tight along the floor.

Zack took aim at the stingers. He sprayed both creatures full in the face—mouth and nose and eyes—before they could get to him. They had a sort of film over their eyes already, and the paint adhered to it, shutting down their vision. They reeled back, trying to clear their eyes with their oversized—for their bodies—hands and having no luck.

This was Zack's chance to pounce and kill—but, knowing more vampires were on the way, he instead picked up his iPod light and ran before the painted vampires perceived him through other senses.

He saw steps and a door stamped with caution signs. It was locked but not bolted, no one expecting burglars this far beneath sea level, and Zack slipped the point of Abraham's blade inside the door crack, working it behind the latch. Inside, the thrum of transformers startled him. He saw no other door, and panicked, thinking he was stuck. But a service duct ran a foot off the floor, out of the wall to the left, before turning and angling into the machinery. Zack chanced a look beneath it and did not see a facing wall. He deliberated a moment, then set his iPod down on the floor, lit-screen up, its light reflecting off the metal bottom of the duct. He then slid it down along beneath the duct like a thin puck gliding over an air hockey table. The up-shining light slid down the floor, turning slightly, but going a long way before stopping, hitting something hard. Zack saw that the light was no longer shining off the reflecting duct.

Zack did not hesitate. He got down on his belly and started beneath the duct before crawling back out again, starting over, realizing he could go faster on his already filthy back. Out he went, headfirst along the narrow crawl space. He slid some fifty feet, the floor at times grabbing his shirt, cutting into his back. At the end, his head popped out into a void, the duct turning and rising high up alongside an embedded ladder.

Zack reclaimed his iPod, shining it up. He could see nothing. But he could hear bumps echoing along the duct: vampire children following his route, moving with preternatural ease.

Zack started up the ladder, his paint can in his hand, Abraham stuck in his belt. He went hand-over-hand up the iron rungs, the echoing duct thumps rising with him. He stopped a moment, hooking his elbow on a rung, pulling the iPod from his pocket to check behind him.

The iPod tumbled from his grip. He grabbed after it, nearly slipping from the ladder, then watched it fall.

As the glowing screen dropped, twisting, it flashed past a form rising up the ladder, illuminating another of his evil playmates.

Zack went back to climbing, faster than he thought he could. But never fast enough. He felt the ladder shaking, and stopped and turned just in time. The child vampire was at his heels when Zack hit it with the paint-can spray, stunning it, blinding it—and then kicking at it with his heel until it fell squealing from the ladder.

He kept climbing, wishing he didn't have to keep looking back. The iPod light was tiny, the floor below a long way away. The ladder shook—harder now. More bodies climbing up the rungs. Zack heard a dog barking—muffled, an exterior noise—and knew he was near some kind of exit.

This gave him a boost of energy and he hurried upward, coming to a flat, round roof.

A manhole. The smooth bottom of it, cold from touching the outside. The surface world was right above. Zack pushed with the heel of his hand. He gave it all he had.

It was no use.

He felt someone near, coming up the ladder, and blindly sprayed the paint below him. He heard a noise like moaning and he kicked downward, but the creature did not fall right away. It was hanging on, swinging. Zack kicked downward with one leg, and a hand grabbed his ankle. A hot hand with a strong grip. A vampire child hanging from him, trying to pull him down. Zack dropped the paint can, needing both hands to grip the ladder. He kicked, trying to ram the creature's fingers into the ladder rungs, but it would not loosen its grip. Until at once—with a squeal—it did.

Zack heard the body smack the wall on the way down.

Another being came up on him before he had time to react. A vampire, he felt its heat, he smelled its earthiness. A hand grabbed his armpit, hooking him, lifting him to the manhole. With two great shoulder shoves, the creature loosened the manhole, throwing it aside. It climbed into the immediate cool of the open air, hauling Zack up with it.

He pulled at the knife at his waist, nearly slicing off his belt trying to work it free. But the vampire's hand closed around his, squeezing hard, holding him there. Zack closed his eyes, not wanting to see the creature. But the grip held him fast and did not move. As though it were waiting.

Zack opened his eyes. He looked up slowly, dreading the sight of its malicious face.

Its eyes were burning red, its hair flat and dead around its face. Its swollen throat bucked, its stinger flicking at the insides of its cheeks. The look it gave him was a mix of vampiric desire and creature satisfaction.

Abraham slipped from Zack's hand.

He said:

"Mom."

They arrived at the building on Central Park via two stolen hotel courtesy cars, encountering no military interference along the way. Inside, the power was out, the elevator inoperable. Gus and the Sapphires started up the stairs, but Setrakian could not climb to the top. Fet did not offer to carry him; Setrakian was too proud for this to even be contemplated. The obstacle appeared insurmountable, and Setrakian, the silver book in his arms, seemed older than ever before.

Fet noted that the elevator was old, with folding gate doors. On a hunch, he went exploring doors near the stairway, and found an old-fashioned dumbwaiter lined with wallpaper. Without a word of protest, Setrakian handed Fet his walking stick and climbed into the half-sized car, sitting with the book on his knees. Angel worked the pulley and counterweight, hauling him up at a gradual rate of speed.

Setrakian rose up in darkness through the building inside the coffin-like conveyance, with his hands resting on the silver plating of the old tome. He was trying to catch his breath, and to settle his mind, but a roll call of sorts ran unbidden through his head: the face of each and every vampire he had ever slain. All the white blood he had spilled, all the worms he had loosed from cursed bodies. For years he had puzzled over the nature of the origin of these monsters on Earth. The Ancients, where they came from. The original act of evil that created these beings.

Fet reached the empty top floor still under construction, and found the door to the dumbwaiter. He opened it and watched a seemingly dazed Setrakian turn and test the floor with his shoe soles before standing out of it. Fet handed him his staff, and the old man blinked and looked at him with only a trace of recognition.

Up a few steps, the door to the empty top-floor apartment was ajar. Gus led the way inside. Mr. Quinlan and a couple of hunters stood beyond the entrance, and only watched them enter. No search, no accosting. Past them, the Ancients stood as before, still as statues, looking out over the falling city.

In absolute silence, Quinlan took position next to a narrow ebony door at the opposite side of the room, wide left of the Ancients. Fet then realized there were only two Ancients now. Where the third had stood, to the far right, all that remained was what appeared to be a pile of white ash in a small wooden urn.

Setrakian walked farther toward them than the hunters had allowed on his previous visit. He stopped near the middle of the room. An illumination flare streaked over Central Park, lighting the apartment and outlining the two remaining Ancients in magnesium-white.

Setrakian said, "So you know."

There was no response.

"Other than Sardu—you were Six Ancients, three Old World, three New. Six birth sites."

Birth is a human act. Six sites of origin.

"One of them was Bulgaria. Then China. But why didn't you safeguard them?"

Hubris, perhaps. Or something quite like it. By the time we knew we were in danger, it was too late. The Young One deceived us. Chernobyl was a decoy—His site. For a long time he managed to stay silent, feeding on carrion. Now he has moved in first—

"Then you know you are doomed."

And then the one on the left vaporized into a burst of fine, white light. His form became dust and fell away to the floor amid a searing noise, like a high-pitched sigh. A shock that was partially electric and partially psychic jolted the humans in the room.

Almost instantaneously, two of the hunters were similarly obliterated. They vanished into a mist finer than smoke, leaving neither ashes nor dust—only their clothes, falling in a warm heap on the floor.

With the Ancient went its sacred bloodline.

The Master was eliminating his only rivals for control of the planet. Was that it?

The irony is that this has always been our plan for the world. Allowing the livestock to erect their own pens, to create and proliferate their weapons and reasons to self-destruct. We have been altering the planet's ecosystem through its master breed. Once the greenhouse effect was irreversible, we were going to reveal ourselves and rise to power.

Setrakian said, "You were making the world over into a vampire nest."

Nuclear winter is a perfect environment. Longer nights, shorter days. We could exist on the surface, shielded from the sun by the contaminated atmosphere. And we were almost there. But he foresaw that. Foresaw that, once we achieved that end, he would have to share with us this planet and its rich food source. And he does not want that.

"What does he want, then?" Setrakian said.

Pain. The Young One wants all the pain he can get. As fast as he can get it. He cannot stop. This addiction . . . this hunger for pain lies, in fact, at the root of our very origin . . .

Setrakian took another step toward the last remaining Ancient. "Quickly. If you are vulnerable through the site of your creation—then so is he."

Now you know what is in the book— You must learn to interpret it . . .

"The location of his origin? Is that it?"

You believed us the ultimate evil. A pox on your people. You thought we were the ultimate corrupters of

your world, and yet we were the glue holding every-
thing together. Now you will feel the lash of the true
overlord.

"Not if you tell us where he is vulnerable—"

We owe you nothing. We are done.

"For revenge, then. He is obliterating you as
you stand here!"

As usual, your human perspective is narrow. The
battle is lost, but nothing is ever obliterated. In any
event, now that he has shown his hand, you may be
certain that he has fortified his earthly place of origin.

"You said Chernobyl," said Setrakian.

Sadum. Amurah.

"What is that? I don't understand," said Setrakian, lifting the book. "If it's here, I am certain.
But I need time to decode it. And we don't have
time."

We were neither born nor created. Sown from an act
of barbarity. A transgression against the high order. An
atrocity. And what was once sown may be reaped.

"How is he different?"

Only stronger. He is like us; we are him—but he is
not us.

In less time than it took to blink, the Ancient
had turned toward him. Its head and face were
time-smoothed, worn of all features, with sagging red eyes, less a nose than a bump, and a
downturned mouth open to toothless blackness.

One thing you must do. Gather every particle of our
remains. Deposit them into a reliquary of silver and
white oak. This is imperative. For us, but also for you.

"Why? Tell me."

White oak. Be certain, Setrakian.

Setrakian said, "I will do no such thing unless I know that doing so won't bring more harm."

You will do it. There is no such thing now as more harm.

Setrakian saw that the Ancient was right.

Fet spoke up behind Setrakian. "We'll collect it—and preserve it in a dustbin."

The Ancient looked past Setrakian for a moment, at the exterminator. With sag-eyed contempt, but also something like pity.

Sadum. Amurah. And his name . . . our name . . .

And then it dawned on Setrakian. "Ozryel . . . The Angel of Death." And he understood everything, and thought all the right questions.

But it was too late.

A blast of white light and a pulse of energy, and the last remaining New World Ancient vanished into a scattering of snow-like ash.

The last remaining hunters twisted as though in a moment of pain—and then evaporated right out of their clothes.

Setrakian felt a breath of ionized air ripple his clothes and fade away.

He sagged, leaning on his staff. The Ancients were no more. And yet a greater evil remained.

In the atomization of the Ancients, he glimpsed his own fate.

Fet was at his side. "What do we do?"

Setrakian found his voice. "Gather the remains."

"You're sure?"

Setrakian nodded. "Use the urn. The reliquary can come later."

He turned and looked for Gus, finding the vampire killer sifting through a hunter's clothes with the tip of his silver sword.

Gus was searching the room for Mr. Quinlan—or his remains—but the Ancients' chief hunter was nowhere to be found.

The narrow door at the left end of the room, however, the ebony door Quinlan had retreated to after they entered, was ajar.

The Ancients' words came back to Gus, from their first meeting:

He is our best hunter. Efficient and loyal. In many respects, unique.

Had Quinlan somehow been spared? Why hadn't he disintegrated like the rest?

"What is it?" asked Setrakian, approaching Gus.

Gus said, "One of the hunters, Quinlan . . . he left no trace . . . Where did he go?"

"It doesn't matter anymore. You are free of them now," said Setrakian. "Free of their control."

Gus looked back at the old man. "Ain't none of us free for long."

"You will have the chance to release your mother."

"If I find her."

"No," said Setrakian. "She will find you."

Gus nodded. "So—nothing's changed."

"One thing. They would have made you one of their hunters if they had succeeded in pushing back the Master. You have been spared that."

"We're splitting," said Creem. "If it's all the same to you. We know the ropes now and it seems to me we can carry on with the good work. But we all have families to gather. Or maybe we don't. Either way, we have places to secure. But if you ever need the Sapphires, Gus—you just come and find us."

Creem shook hands with Gus. Angel stood by uncertainly. He sized up one gang leader, and then the other. He nodded at Gus. The big ex-wrestler had chosen to stay.

Gus turned to Setrakian. "I'm one of your hunters now."

Setrakian said, "You don't need anything more from me. But I need one more thing from you."

"Just name it."

"A ride. A fast one."

"Fast is my specialty. They got more Hummers in a garage underneath this funhouse. Unless that shit evaporated too."

Gus went off to claim a vehicle. Fet had located, inside a chest of drawers in an adjoining room, a briefcase full of cash. He dumped out the paper currency so that Angel had something to deposit the Ancients' ashes in. He had heard the entire conversation with Gus. "I think I know where we are going."

"No," said Setrakian, still looking distracted, only half-there. "Just me." He handed Fet the *Occido Lumen* and his notebook.

"I don't want this," said Fet.

"You must take it. And remember. *Sadum, Amurah.* Will you remember that, Vasiliy?"

"I don't need to remember anything—I'm going with you."

"No. The book is the thing now. It must be kept safe, and out of the Master's claws. We can't lose it now."

"We can't lose you."

Setrakian shook that off. "I am very nearly lost as it is."

"That's why you need me with you."

"*Sadum. Amurah.* Say it," said Setrakian. "That's what you can do for me. Let me hear that—let me know that you keep those words . . ."

"*Sadum. Amurah,*" said Fet obediently. "I know them."

Setrakian nodded. "This world is going to become a terribly hard place of little hope. Protect those words—that book—like a flame. Read it. The key to it is in my notes. Their nature, their origin, their name—they were all one . . ."

"You know I can't make heads or tails—"

"Then go to Ephraim, together you will. You must go to him now." His voice broke. "You two need to stay together."

"Two of us together doesn't equal one of you. Give this to Gus. Let me take you, please . . ." Now there were tears in the eyes of the exterminator.

Setrakian's gnarled hand gripped Fet's forearm with fading strength. "It is your responsibility now, Vasiliy. I trust you implicitly . . . Be bold."

The silver plating was cold to touch. He accepted the book finally, because the old man insisted, like a dying man pressing his diary into the hands of a reluctant heir. "What are you going to do?" asked Fet, knowing now that this was the last time he would see Setrakian. "What can you do?"

Setrakian released Fet's arm. "One thing only, my son."

It was that word—"son"—that touched Fet the deepest. He choked back his pain as he watched the old man move along.

The mile Eph ran into the North River Tunnel felt like ten. Guided only by Fet's night-vision monocular, over a glowing green landscape of unchanging train tracks, Eph's descent beneath the Hudson River was a true journey into madness. Dizzied and frantic, and gasping for breath, he began to see glowing white stains along the rail ties.

He slowed long enough to pull a Luma lamp from the pack on his back. The ultraviolet light picked up an explosion of color, the biological matter expelled by vampires. The staining was recent, the ammonia odor eye-watering. This much waste indicated a massive feeding.

Eph ran until he saw the rear car of the derailed train. No noise; all was still. Eph started around the right, seeing ahead where the engine or the first passenger car had jumped the track, angled up against the tunnel wall. He entered an open door, boarding the dark train. Through his green vision, he viewed the carnage. Bodies slumped over chairs, over other bodies, on the floor. All budding vampires, due to begin rising as soon as the next sunset. No time to release them all now. Or to go through them, face-by-face.

No. He knew Nora was smarter than that.

He jumped back out, turning the corner around the train, and saw the lurkers. Four of them, two to a side, their eyes reflecting like glass in his monocular. His Luma lamp froze them, hungry faces leering as they backed away, allowing him passage.

Eph knew better. He went between the two pairs, counting to three before reaching back and drawing his sword from his pack, and wheeling around.

He caught them coming, slashing the first two aggressors, then going after the backpedalers and cutting them down without hesitation.

Before their bodies settled on the tracks, Eph returned to the wet trail of vampire waste. It led to a passage through the left wall, into the facing, Manhattan-bound track. Eph followed the swirling colors, ignoring his disgust, rushing through the dark tunnel. He passed two hacked corpses—the bright register of their spilled blood under the black light showing them to be *strigoi*—then heard a ruckus ahead.

He came upon some nine or ten creatures bunched up at a door. They fanned out upon sensing him, Eph sweeping his Luma lamp in order to prevent any from slipping behind him.

The door. Zack was inside, Eph told himself.

He went homicidal, attacking before the vampires could coordinate an assault. Slashing and burning. His animal brutality surpassed theirs.

His paternal need overmatched their blood hunger. This was a fight for his son's life, and for a father pushed to the brink, killing came quick. Killing was easy.

He went to the door, clanging his white-slickened sword blade against it. "Zack! It's me! Open up!"

The hand holding the door fast from the inside released the knob, Eph ripping open the door. There stood Nora, her wide eyes as bright as the flare burning in her hand. She stared at him a long moment, as though making sure it was him—a human him—then rushed into his arms. Behind her, sitting on a box in her house-coat with her gaze cast sadly into the corner, was Nora's mother.

Eph closed his arms around Nora as best he could without letting the wet blade touch her. Then, realizing the rest of the storage closet was empty, he pushed back.

"Where's Zack?" he said.

Gus blew through the open perimeter gate, the dark silhouettes of the cooling towers looming in the distance. Motion-sensitive surveillance cameras sat on high white poles like heads upon pikes, failing to track their Hummer as it passed. The road in was long and winding, and they were unmet.

Setrakian rode in the passenger seat with his hand over his heart. High fences topped with barbwire; towers spewing smokelike steam. A camp flashback rippled through him like nausea.

"Federales," said Angel, from the backseat.

National Guard trucks were set up at the entrance to the interior security zone. Gus slowed, awaiting some signal or order that he would then have to figure out a way to disobey.

When no such order came, he rolled right up to the gate and stopped. He exited the Hummer with the engine running, checking the first truck. Empty. The second as well. Empty but for splashes of red blood on the windshield and dashboard, and a dry puddle on the front seat.

Gus went into the back of the truck, lifting the canvas. He waved over Angel, who came limping. Together they looked at the rack of small arms. Angel strung one submachine gun over each of his considerable shoulders, cradling an assault rifle in his arms. Extra ammunition went into his pockets and shirt. Gus carried two Colt submachine guns back to the Hummer.

They pushed around the trucks through to the first buildings. Getting out, Setrakian heard loud engines running and realized the plant was operating on diesel-fueled backup generators. The redundant safety systems were operating automatically, keeping the abandoned reactor from shutting down.

Inside the first buildings, they were met by turned soldiers—vampires in fatigues. With Gus in front and Angel limping behind, they moved through the revenants, shredding bodies without any finesse. The rounds staggered the vampires, but they wouldn't stay down unless the spinal column was obliterated at the neck.

"Know where you're going?" said Gus over his shoulder.

"I do not," said Setrakian.

He followed the security checkpoints, pushing through doors with the most warning signs. Here there were no more soldier vampires, only plant workers turned into guards and sentinels. The more resistance Setrakian met, the closer he knew they were to the control room.

Setrakian.

The old man grabbed the wall.

The Master. Here . . .

How much more powerful the Master's "voice" was inside his head than that of the Ancients. Like a hand grasping his brain stem and snapping his spine like a whip.

Angel straightened Setrakian with a meaty hand and called to Gus.

"What is it?" said Gus, fearing a heart attack.

They hadn't heard it. The Master spoke only to Setrakian.

"He is here now," said Setrakian. "The Master."

Gus looked this way and that, hyperalert. "He's here? Great. Let's get him."

"No. You don't understand. You haven't faced him yet. He is not like the Ancients. These guns are nothing to him. He will dance around bullets."

Gus reloaded his smoking weapon and said, "I come too far with this. Nothing scares me now."

"I know, but you can't beat him this way. Not here, and not with weapons made for killing men." Setrakian fixed his vest, straightening. "I know what he wants."

"Okay. What's that?"

"Something only I can give him."

"That damn book?"

"No. Listen to me, Gus. Return to Manhattan. If you leave now, there is hope that you might make it in time. Join Eph and Fet if you can. You will need to be deep underground regardless."

"This place is going to blow?" Gus looked at Angel, who was breathing hard and gripping his bad leg. "Then come back with us. Let's go. If you can't beat him here."

"I can't stop this nuclear chain reaction. But—I might be able to affect the chain reaction of vampiric infection."

An alarm went off—piercing honks spaced about one second apart—startling Angel, who checked both ends of the hallway.

"My guess is the backup generators are failing," said Setrakian. He grasped Gus's shirt, talking over the horn blasts. "Do you want to be cooked alive here? Both of you—go!"

Gus remained with Angel as the old man walked on, unsheathing the sword from his walking stick. Gus looked to the other old man in his charge, the broken-down wrestler drenched in sweat, his big eyes uncertain. Waiting to be told what to do.

"We go," said Gus. "You heard the man."

Angel's big arm stopped him. "Just leave him here?"

Gus shook his head hard, knowing there was no good solution. "I'm only alive still because of him. For me, whatever the pawnbroker says, goes. Now let's get as far away from here as we can, unless you want to see your own skeleton."

Angel was still looking after Setrakian, and had to be pulled away by Gus.

Setrakian entered the control room and saw a lone creature in an old suit standing before a series of panels, watching gauge dials roll back as systems failed. Red emergency lights flashed from every corner of the room, though the alarm was muted.

Eichhorst turned just its head, red eyes settling on its former camp prisoner. No concern in his face—it wasn't capable of the subtleties of emotion, and barely registered the larger reactions, such as surprise.

You are just in time, it said, returning to the monitors.

Setrakian, sword at his side, circled behind the creature.

I don't believe I extended you my congratulations on winning the book. That was a clever bit of work, going around Palmer like that.

"I expected to meet him here."

You won't be seeing him again. He never realized his great dream, precisely because he failed to understand that it was not his aspirations that mattered but the Master's. You creatures and your pathetic hopes.

Setrakian said, "Why you? Why did he keep you?"

The Master learns from humans. That is a key element of his greatness. He watches and he sees. Your kind has shown him the way to your own final solution. I see only packs of animals, but he sees patterns of behavior. He listens to what you are saying when, as I suspect, you have no idea you are saying anything at all.

"You're saying he learned from you? Learned what?" Setrakian's grip tightened on the handle of his sword as Eichhorst turned. He looked at the former camp commandant—and suddenly he knew.

It is not easy to establish and operate a well-functioning camp. It took a special kind of human intellect to oversee the systematic destruction of a people at maximum efficiency. He drew upon my singular knowledge.

Setrakian went dry. He felt as though his flesh were crumbling off his bones.

Camps. Human stockyards. Blood farms spread out across the country, the world.

In a sense, Setrakian had always known. Always known but never wanted to believe. He had seen it in the Master's eyes upon their first meeting in the barracks at Treblinka. Man's own inhumanity to man had whet the monster's appetite for havoc. We had, through our atrocities, demonstrated our own doom to the ultimate nemesis, welcoming him as though by prophesy.

The building shuddered as a bank of monitors went dark.

Setrakian cleared his throat to find his voice. "Where is your Master now?"

He is everywhere, don't you know? Here, now. Watching you. Through me.

Setrakian readied himself, taking a step forward. His course was clear. "He must be pleased with your handiwork. But he has little use for you now. No more than I do."

You underestimate me, Jew.

Eichhorst vaulted up onto the nearby console with little apparent effort, moving out of Setrakian's kill range. Setrakian raised his silver blade, its tip pointing at the Nazi's throat. Eichhorst's arms were at his sides, elongated fingers rubbing against his palms. It feigned an attack; Setrakian countering but not giving any quarter. The old vampire leaped to another console, shoes trampling on the tender controls of this highly sensitive room. Setrakian swung around, tracking it—until he faltered.

With the hand holding the wooden sheath of his walking stick, Setrakian pressed his crooked knuckles to his chest, over his heart.

Your pulse is most irregular.

Setrakian winced and staggered. He exaggerated his distress, but not for Eichhorst's sake. His sword arm bent, but he kept the blade high.

Eichhorst hopped down to the floor, watching Setrakian with something like nostalgia.

I no longer know the tether of the heartbeat. The lung breath. The cheap gear-work and slow tick of the human clock.

Setrakian leaned against the console. Waiting for strength to return.

And you would rather perish than continue on in a greater form?

Setrakian said, "Better to die a man than live as a monster."

Can you fail to see that, to all the lesser beings, you are the monster? It is you who took this planet for your own. And now the worm turns.

Eichhorst's eyes flickered a moment, their nictitating lids narrowing.

He commands me to turn you. I do not look forward to your blood. Hebraic inbreeding has fortified the bloodline into a vintage as salty and mineral-muddied as the River Jordan.

"You won't turn me. The Master himself couldn't turn me."

Eichhorst moved laterally, not yet attempting to close the distance between them.

Your wife struggled but she never cried out. I thought that strange. Not even a whimper. Only a single word. "Abraham."

Setrakian allowed himself to be goaded, wanting the vampire closer. "She saw the end. She found solace in the moment, knowing that I would someday avenge her."

She called your name and you were not there. I wonder if you will sing out at the end.

Setrakian sank almost to one knee before lowering his blade, using the point against the floor as a kind of crutch, to keep himself from falling.

Put aside your weapon, Jew.

Setrakian lifted his sword, switching to an

overhand grip of the handle in order to examine the line of the old silver blade. He looked at the wolf's head pommel, feeling its counterbalancing weight.

Accept your fate.

"Ah," said Setrakian, looking at Eichhorst standing just a few feet away. "But I already have."

Setrakian put everything he had into the throw. The sword crossed the space between them and penetrated Eichhorst just below the breastplate, dead-center in his torso, between the buttons of his vest. The vampire fell back against the console with his bent arms back as though in a gesture of balance. The killing silver was in his body and he could not touch it to pull out the blade. He began to twitch as the silver's toxic virucidal properties spread outward like a burning cancer. White blood appeared around the blade with the first of the escaping worms.

Setrakian pulled himself to his feet and stood, wavering, before Eichhorst. He did so with no sense of triumph, and little satisfaction. He made certain that the vampire's eyes were focused on him—and, by extension, the Master's eyes—and said, "Through him you took love away from me. Now you will have to turn me yourself." Then he grasped the sword handle and slowly pulled it from Eichhorst's chest.

The vampire settled back against the console, its hands still grasping at nothing. It began to slide to the right, falling stiffly, and Setrakian, in his weakened state, anticipated Eichhorst's trajectory and set the point of his sword against the floor. The blade rested at about a forty-degree angle, the angle of the guillotine blade.

Eichhorst's falling body pulled its neck across the edge of the blade, and the Nazi was destroyed.

Setrakian swiped both sides of his silver blade over the vampire's coat sleeve, cleaning them, then backed away from the blood worms fleeing Eichhorst's open neck. His chest seized up like a knot. He reached for his pillbox and, in trying to open it with his twisted hands, spilled the contents onto the control-room floor.

Gus emerged from the nuke plant ahead of Angel, into the dim, overcast last day. Between the persistent alarm blasts, he heard a deathly silence, the generators no longer working. He sensed a low-voltage snap in the air, like static electricity, but it might just have been him knowing what was to come.

Then, a familiar noise cutting into the air. A helicopter. Gus found the lights, seeing the chopper circle behind the steaming towers. He knew it wasn't help on the way. He realized that this had to be the Master's ride out of here, so it didn't cook with the rest of Long Island.

Gus went into the back of the National Guard truck. He had seen the Stinger missile the first time, but stuck with the small arms. All he needed was a reason.

He brought it out and double-checked to make sure he had it facing the right way. It balanced nicely on his shoulder and was surprisingly light for an antiaircraft weapon, maybe thirty-five pounds. He ran past the limping Angel to the side of the building. The chopper was coming in lower, making to land in a wide clearing.

The trigger was easy to find, as was the scope. He looked through it, and once the missile detected the heat of the helicopter's exhaust, it emitted a high, whistle-like tone. Gus squeezed the trigger and the launch rocket shot the missile out of the tube. The launch engine fell away and the main solid rocket engine lit up and the Stinger flew off like a plume of smoke traveling along a string.

The helicopter never saw it coming. The missile struck it a few hundred yards above the ground and the flying machine burst upon impact, the explosion upending it and sending it pinwheeling into nearby trees.

Gus threw off the empty launcher. The fire was good. It would light his way to the water. Long Island Sound was the fastest and safest way back home.

He said as much to Angel, but he could tell, as the distant light of the flames played across the old brawler's face, that something had changed.

"I'm staying," said Angel.

Gus tried to explain that which he only vaguely understood himself. "This whole place is going to go up. This is nukes."

"I can't walk away from a fight." Angel patted his leg to show that he meant it literally as well as figuratively. "Besides, I've been here before."

"Here?"

"In my movies. I know how it ends. The evil one faces the good one, and all seems lost."

"Angel," said Gus, needing to go.

"The day is saved always—in the end."

Gus had noticed the ex-wrestler acting more and more scattered. The vampire siege was wearing on his mind, his perspective. "Not here. Not against this."

Angel pulled, from deep in his front pocket, a piece of cloth. He pulled it on over his head, rolling the silver mask down so that only his eyes and his mouth showed. "You go," he said. "Back to the island, with the doctor. Do as the old man tell you. Me? He have no plan for me. So I stay. I fight."

Gus smiled at the mad Mexican's bravery. And he recognized Angel for the very first time. He understood everything—the strength, the courage of this old man. As a child, he had seen all of the wrestler's films on TV. On weekends, they played on an endless loop. And now he was standing next to his hero. "This world is a motherfucker, isn't it?"

Angel nodded and said, "But it's the only one we have."

Gus felt a surge of love for this fucked-up fellow countryman. For his matinee idol. His eyes welled up as he clapped his hands against the big man's shoulders. He said, *"Que viva el Ángel de Plata, culeros!"*

Angel nodded. *"Que viva!"*

And with that, the Silver Angel turned back, limping, toward the doomed power plant.

                              *   *   *

Emergency lights flashed, the exterior alarm muted inside the control room. The wall panel instruments blinked, imploring human hands to take action.

Setrakian knelt on the floor across from Eichhorst's still body. Eichhorst's head had rolled almost to the corner. One of Setrakian's pocket mirrors had cracked, and he was using the silver back to crush the blood worms seeking him out. With his other hand, he was trying to pick up his heart pills, but his gnarled fingers and arthritic knuckles had trouble with the pincer grip.

And then he was aware of a presence, whose sudden arrival changed the atmosphere of the already charged room. No puff of smoke, no crack of thunder. A psychic blow more breathtaking than mere stagecraft. Setrakian didn't have to look up to know it was the Master—and yet he did look up, from the hem of its dark cloak to its imperious face.

Its flesh had peeled back to the sub-dermis, save for a few patches of sun-cooked skin. A fiery red beast with splotches of black. Its eyes roared with intensity, a bloodier hue of red. The circulating worms rippled beneath the surface like twitching nerves alive with madness.

It is done.

The Master seized the wolf's-head handle of Setrakian's sword before the old man could react. The creature held the silver blade for inspection the way a man might handle a glowing-hot poker.

The world is mine.

The Master, his movement no more than a blur, retrieved the wooden sheath from the floor on the other side of Setrakian. He fit the two pieces together, burying the blade inside the cavity of the original walking stick and fixing the joined staff with a sudden wrenching twist of his hands.

Then he returned the foot of the stick to the floor. The overlong walking stick was a perfect fit, of course: it had belonged to the human giant Sardu, in whose body the Master currently resided.

The nuclear fuel inside the reactor core is beginning to overheat and melt. This facility was constructed using modern safeguards, but the automatic containment procedures only delay the inevitable. The meltdown will occur, fouling and destroying this origin site of the sixth and only remaining member of my clan. The buildup of steam will result in a catastrophic reactor explosion that will release a plume of radioactive fallout.

The Master jabbed Setrakian in the ribs with the end of the walking stick, the old man hearing and feeling a crack, curling into a ball on the floor.

As my shadow falls over you, Setrakian, so does it fall over this planet. First I infected your people, now I have infected the globe. Your half-dark world was not enough. How long I have looked forward to this permanent, lasting dusk. This warm, blue-green rock shivers at my touch, becoming a cold black stone of rime and rot. The sunset of humankind is the dawn of the blood harvest.

The Master's head then turned a few degrees, toward the door. He was not alarmed, nor even annoyed, more like curious. Setrakian turned also, a sizzle of hope rising along his back. The door opened and Angel entered limping, wearing a mask of shiny silver nylon with black stitching.

"No," gasped Setrakian.

Angel carried an automatic weapon, and, seeing the eight-foot-tall cloaked creature towering over Setrakian, opened up on the king vampire.

The creature stood there for a moment, gazing at its patently ridiculous opponent. But as the bullets flew, the Master became, instinctively, a blur—the rounds carrying across the room into the sensitive equipment lining the walls. The Master paused on one side of the room, visible for just the briefest moment, though by the time Angel turned and fired, the vampire was moving again. The rounds ripped into a control panel, sparks shooting out of the wall.

Setrakian returned his attention to the floor, frantically picking at the tiny pills.

The Master slowed again, with the effect of materializing before Angel. The masked wrestler dropped the big gun with a clatter and lunged at the creature.

The Master noted the big human's weak knee, but those things could be fixed. The body was aged, yet size-appropriate. Suitable, perhaps, for temporary housing.

The Master eluded Angel. The wrestler swung around, but the Master was already behind him again. While assessing Angel, the Master slapped him on the back of his neck, where the stitched hem of his mask met skin. The wrestler jerked around wildly again.

Angel was being toyed with, and he didn't like it. He turned fast and came around with his free hand, catching the Master on the chin with an open-palm blow. The "Angel Kiss."

The creature's head snapped back. Angel shocked himself with his success in landing the blow. The Master lowered his eyes at the masked avenger, the speed of the worms rippling under his flesh a sign of his rage.

Inside the mask, Angel smiled excitedly.

"You would like me to reveal myself, wouldn't you?" he said. "The mystery dies with me. My face must remain hidden."

These words were the catchphrase from every one of the Silver Angel's movies, dubbed into many languages all over the world—words the wrestler had been waiting for decades to say for real. But the Master was through playing.

It struck Angel full-force with the back of its enormous hand. The jaw and left cheekbone exploded inside the mask and the wrestler's left eye went with them.

But Angel didn't give up. Through enormous effort, he stood on his own two feet. Trembling, his knee hurting like a motherfucker, choking on his own blood . . . yet in his mind he raced back in time, to a younger, happier place.

He felt dizzy and warm and full of juice and remembered he was in a film stage. Of course—he was shooting a movie. The monster in front of him was nothing but some clever special effect—a day player in a suit. Then why did it hurt so much? And his mask: it smelled funny to him. Like unwashed hair and sweat. It smelled like a thing removed to the oblivion of storage. It smelled of him.

An empty bubble of blood rose in his throat and burst there in a liquid whimper. His jaw and left side pulverized, the smelly mask was now the only thing holding the old wrestler's face together.

Angel grunted and lunged at his opponent. The Master released the stick in order to grip the big human with both hands, and, in an instant, tore him to shreds.

Setrakian stifled a cry. He was stuffing pills in under his tongue—stopping just as the Master returned his attention to him.

The Master grasped Setrakian's shoulder and lifted the slight old man off the floor. Setrakian dangled in the air before the Master, squeezed by the vampire's bloody hands. The Master pulled him close, Setrakian staring into its horrible face, the leech's face swarming with ancient evil.

I believe, in a way, you always wanted this, Professor. I think you have always been curious to know the other side.

Setrakian could not respond with the pills dissolving beneath his tongue. But he did not have to answer the Master verbally. *My sword sings of silver,* he thought.

He felt woozy, the medicine kicking in, clouding his thoughts—shielding his true intent from the Master's perception. *We learned much from the book. We know Chernobyl was a decoy . . .* He saw the

Master's face. How he longed to see fear in it. *Your name. I know your true name. Would you like to hear it . . . Ozryel?*

And then the Master's mouth fell open and his stinger shot out furiously, snapping and piercing Setrakian's neck, rupturing his vocal cords and jamming into his carotid artery. As he lost his voice, Setrakian felt no stinging pain, only the body-wide ache of the drinking. The collapse of his circulatory system and the organs it served, leading to shock.

The Master's eyes were royal-red, staring at its prey's face as it drank with immense satisfaction. Setrakian held the creature's gaze, not out of defiance but watching and waiting for some indication of discomfort. He felt the vibration of the blood worms wriggling throughout his body, greedily inspecting and invading his self.

All at once, the Master bucked, as though choking. His head jerked back and his nictitating eyelids fluttered. Still, the seal remained tight, the drinking continued stubbornly until the end. The Master disengaged finally—the entire process having taken less than half a minute—its flushed red stinger retracting. The Master stared at Setrakian, reading the interest in his eyes, then stumbled backward a step. Its face contracted, the blood worms slowing, its thick neck gagging.

It dropped Setrakian to the floor and staggered away, sickened by the old man's blood meal. A flame-like sensation in the pit of his gut.

Setrakian lay on the floor of the control room in a dim haze, bleeding through the puncture wound. He finally relaxed his tongue, feeling that the last of the pills in the basket of his jaw were gone. He had ingested the blood vessel–relaxing nitroglycerin and the blood-thinning Coumadin derivative of Fet's rat poison in massive overdose levels, and passed them along to the Master.

Fet was, indeed, correct: the creatures had no purging mechanism. Once a substance was ingested, they could not vomit it.

Burning inside, the Master moved through the doors at a blur, racing off into the screaming alarms.

The Johnson Space Center went silent halfway through the station's dark orbit, as they passed the dark side of the Earth. She'd lost Houston.

Thalia felt the first few bumps shortly after that. It was debris, space junk plunking the station. Nothing very unusual about that—only the frequency of the impacts.

Too many. Too close together.

She floated as still as possible, trying to calm herself, trying to think. Something wasn't right.

She made her way to the porthole and gazed out upon the Earth. Two very hot points of light were visible here on the night side of the planet. One was on the very edge, right on the ridge of dusk. Another one was nearer to the eastern side.

She had never witnessed anything like it, and nothing in her training or the many manuals she had read prepared her for this sight. The intensity of the light, its evident heat—mere pinpoints on the globe itself, and yet her trained eye knew that these were explosions of enormous magnitude.

The station was rocked by another firm impact. This was not the usual small metal hail of space debris. An emergency indicator went off, yellow lights flashing near the door. Something had perforated the solar panels. It was as though the space station were under fire. Now she would need to suit up and—

BAMMM! Something had struck the hull. She swam over to a computer and saw immediately the warning of an oxygen leak. A rapid one. The tanks had been perforated. She called out to her shipmates, heading for the airlock.

A bigger impact shook the hull. Thalia suited up as fast as she could, but the station itself had been breached. She struggled to fasten her suit helmet, racing the deadly vacuum. With her last ounce of strength, she opened the oxygen valve.

Thalia drifted into darkness, losing consciousness. Her final thought before blackout was not of her husband but of her dog. In the silence of space, she somehow heard him barking.

Soon the International Space Station joined the rest of the flotsam hurtling through space, gradually slipping from its orbit, floating inexorably toward Earth.

Setrakian's head swam as he lay on the floor of the rumbling Locust Valley Nuclear Power Plant.

He was turning. He could feel it.

A constricting pain in his throat that was only the beginning. His chest a hive of activity. The blood worms had settled and released their payload: the virus breeding quickly inside him, overwhelming his cells. Changing him. Trying to remake him.

His body could not withstand the turning. Even without his now-weakened veins, he was too old, too weak. He was like a thin-stemmed sunflower bending under the weight of its growing head. Or a fetus growing from bad chromosomes.

The voices. He heard them. The buzz of a greater consciousness. A coordination of being. A concert of cacophony.

He felt heat. From his rising body temperature, but also from the trembling floor. The cooling system meant to prevent hot nuclear fuel from melting had failed—failed on purpose. The fuel had melted through the bottom of the reactor core. Once it reached the water table, the ground beneath the plant would erupt in a lethal release of steam.

Setrakian.

The Master's voice in his head. Phasing in and out with his own. Setrakian had a vision then, of what looked like the rear of a truck—the National Guard trucks he had seen outside the plant's entrance. The view from the floor, vague and monochromatic, seen through the eyes of a being with night vision enhanced beyond human ability.

Setrakian saw his walking stick—Sardu's walking stick—rattling around just a few feet away, as though he could reach out and touch it one last time.

Pic—pic—pic . . .

He was seeing what the Master saw.

Setrakian, you fool.

The floor of the truck rumbled, speeding away. The view rocked back and forth as though seen by a thing writhing in pain.

You thought poisoning your blood could kill me?

Setrakian pulled himself up onto all fours, relying on the temporary strength the turning imbued him with.

Pic—pic . . .

I have sickened you, strigoi, Setrakian thought. *Again I have weakened you.*

And he knew the Master could hear him now.

You are turned.

I have finally released Sardu. And soon I will be released myself.

And he said nothing more, the nascent vampire Setrakian dragging himself closer to the endangered core.

Pressure continued to build inside the containment structure. A bubble of toxic hydrogen expanding out of control. The steel-reinforced concrete shield would only make the ultimate explosion worse.

Setrakian pulled himself arm by arm, leg by leg. His body turning inside, his mind aflutter with the sight of a thousand eyes, his head singing with the chorus of a thousand voices.

Zero hour was at hand. They were all heading underground.

Pic . . .

"Silence, *strigoi.*"

Then the nuclear fuel reached the groundwater. The earth beneath the plant erupted, and the origin place of the final Ancient was obliterated— as was Setrakian, in the same instant.

No more.

The pressure vessel cracked open and released a radioactive cloud over Long Island Sound.

Gabriel Bolivar, the former rock star and the only remaining member of the original four Regis Air survivors, waited deep beneath the meatpacking plant. It had been called upon especially by the Master, called to be ready.

Gabriel, my child.

The voices hummed, droning as one in perfect fidelity. The old man, Setrakian—his voice had been silenced forever.

Gabriel. The name of an archangel . . . So appropriate . . .

Bolivar awaited the dark father, feeling him near. Knowing of his victory on the surface. All that was left now was to wait for the new world to set and cure.

The Master entered the black dirt chamber. The Master stood before Bolivar, its head crooked at the chamber ceiling. Bolivar could feel the Master's body distress, but its mind—its word— sang as true as ever.

In me, you will live. In my hunger and my voice and my breath—and we will live in you. Our minds will reside in yours and our blood will race together.

The Master threw off its cloak, reaching its long arm into its coffin, scooping out a handful of rich soil. He fed it into Bolivar's unswallowing mouth.

And you will be my son and I your father and we will rule as I and us, forever.

The Master clutched Bolivar in a great embrace. Bolivar was alarmingly thin, appearing fragile and small against the Master's colossal frame. Bolivar felt swallowed, possessed. He felt received. For the first time in life or death, Gabriel Bolivar felt at home.

The worms came spilling out of the Master, hundreds and hundreds of them, seeping out of its reddened flesh. The frenzied worms wove all around them, in and out of their flesh, fusing the two beings in a crimson embroidery.

Then, finally, the Master released the old husk of the long-ago giant, which crumbled and broke away as it hit the floor. And, as he did so, the soul of the boy-hunter also found release. It disappeared from the chorus of voices, the hymn that animated the Master.

Sardu was no more. Gabriel Bolivar was something new.

Bolivar/the Master spit the soil out. It opened its mouth and tested its stinger. The fleshy protuberance rode out with a firm snap, and recoiled.

The Master was reborn.

The body was unfamiliar somehow, the Master

having been accustomed to Sardu for so long, but this transitional body was flexible and fresh. The Master would soon put it to the test.

At any rate, this human physicality was of little concern to the Master now. The giant's body had suited the creature when it lived among the shadows. But size and durability of the host body mattered little now. Not in this new world that it had created in its own image.

The Master sensed human intrusion. A strong heart, a swift pulse. A boy.

Out of the adjoining tunnel, Kelly Goodweather arrived with her son, Zachary, firmly in her grip. The boy stood trembling, crouched over in a posture of self-protection. He saw nothing in the darkness, only sensing presences, heated bodies in the cool underground. He smelled ammonia and dank soil and something rotting.

Kelly approached with the pride of a cat depositing a mouse at its master's threshold. The Master's physical appearance, revealed to her night-seeing eyes in the blackness of the underground chamber, did not confound her in the least. She saw his presence within Bolivar and questioned nothing.

The Master scraped some magnesium from the wall, sprinkling it into the basket of a torch. He then chipped into the stone with his long middle nail, a spray of sparks igniting the small torch, bringing an orange glow to the chamber.

Zack saw before him a bony vampire with glowing red eyes and a slack expression. His mind had mostly shut down in panic, but there was still that small part of him that trusted his mother, that found calm so long as she was near.

Then, near the gaunt vampire, Zack saw the empty corpse lying on the floor, its sun-damaged, vinyl-smooth flesh still glistening. The creature's pelt.

He saw also a walking stick leaning against the cave wall. The wolf's head caught the flicker of the flame.

Professor Setrakian.

No.

Yes.

The voice was inside his head. Answering him with the power and authority Zack suspected God might speak to him someday, in answer to his prayers.

But this was not God's voice. This was the commanding presence of the thin creature before him.

"Dad," Zack whispered. His father had been with the professor. Tears welled up. "Dad."

Zack's mouth moved, but the word had no breath behind it. His lungs were locking up. He felt his pockets for his inhaler. His knees buckling, Zack slumped to the ground.

Kelly watched her suffering son impassively. The Master had been prepared to destroy Kelly. The Master was unaccustomed to defiance, and could think of no reason why Kelly had not turned the boy immediately.

Now the Master saw why. Kelly's bond with the boy was so strong, the affection so potent, that she had instead brought him to the Master to be turned.

This was an act of devotion. An offering borne out of the human precursor—love—to vampire need, which, in fact, surpassed that need.

And the Master did indeed hunger. And the boy was a fine specimen. He would be honored to receive the Master.

But now . . . things appeared different in the darkness of a new night.

The Master saw more benefit in waiting.

It sensed the distress in the boy's chest, his heart first racing, and now starting to slow. The boy lay on the ground, clutching at his throat, the Master standing over him. The Master pricked its thumb with the sharp nail of its prominent middle finger, and, taking care not to let slip any worms, allowed one single white drop to fall into the boy's open mouth, landing upon his gasping tongue.

The boy groaned suddenly, sucking air. In his mouth, the taste of copper and hot camphor—but in a few moments, he was breathing normally again. Once, on a dare, Zack had licked the ends of a nine-volt battery. That was the jolt he had felt before his lungs opened. He looked up at the Master—this creature, this presence—with the awe of the cured.

EPILOGUE

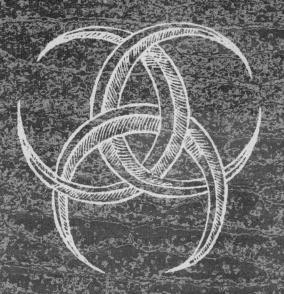

Extract from the diary of Ephraim Goodweather

Sunday, November 28

With every city and province around the globe—already alarmed by initial reports out of New York City—now afflicted by growing waves of unexplained disappearances . . .

With rumors and wild tales—of the vanished returning to their homes after dark, possessed of inhuman desires—spreading at speeds more scorching than the pandemic itself . . .

With terms like "vampirism" and "plague" finally being uttered by those in positions of power and influence . . .

And with the economy, the media, and transportation systems all failing throughout the globe . . .

. . . the world had already teetered over the edge, into full-blown panic.

And then began the nuclear-plant meltdowns. One after the other.

No official sequence of events or proper time line can, nor ever will be, verified, due to the mass destruction and subsequent devastation. What follows is the accepted hypothesis, though admittedly a "best guess" based mainly upon the arrangement of the tiles before the first domino fell.

After China, the reactor failure of a Stoneheart-constructed nuclear plant in Hadera, on the western coast of Israel, led to a second core meltdown. A vapor cloud of radioactivity was released, containing large particles of radioisotopes as well as caesium and tellurium in aerosol form. Warm Mediterranean wind currents scattered the contamination northeast into Syria and Turkey and over the Black Sea into Russia, as well as east over Iraq and northern Iran.

Terrorist sabotage was suspected as the cause, with fingers pointed at Pakistan. Pakistan denied any involvement, while a meeting of the Israeli cabinet followed an emergency meeting of the Knesset, viewed as a war council. Meanwhile, Syria and Cyprus demanded international censure of Israel as well as financial reparations, and Iran declared that the vampire curse was also obviously Jewish in origin.

Pakistan's president and prime minister, believing that the reactor meltdown was an excuse for Israel to launch an attack, led the parliament to authorize a preemptive nuclear strike of six warheads.

Israel countered with their second strike capability.

Iran bombed Israel and immediately claimed

*victory. India launched retaliatory fifteen-kiloton
warheads against Pakistan and Iran.*

*North Korea, spurred on by fear of the plague as
well as an extended famine, launched against South
Korea and sent its troops across the thirty-eighth
parallel.*

*China allowed itself to be drawn into the conflict,
in an attempt to distract the international community
from its own catastrophic nuclear reactor failure.*

*The nuclear explosions triggered earthquakes
and volcanic eruptions. Tons and tons of ash were
injected into the stratosphere, along with sulfuric
acid and massive amounts of greenhouse gas carbon
dioxide.*

*Cities burned and oil fields ignited, consuming
many million barrels of oil daily, fires that could not
be extinguished by man. These continuous chimneys
lofted dark, blanketing smoke into the ash-saturated
stratosphere, cycling over the planet, absorbing
sunlight at levels reaching 80 to 90 percent.*

This cooling soot grew like a cowl over the Earth.

*It impacted every human settlement, bringing
further chaos and the certainty of the Rapture. Cities
degenerated into toxic prisons, highways became
gridlocked junkyards. The Canadian and Mexican
borders were closed and illegal U.S. citizens crossing
the Rio Grande were met with decisive firepower.
Though even these boundaries were not to last.*

*Above Manhattan, the massive radioactive
cloud lingered, the sky turning crimson until the
atmospheric soot blotted out the sun. The dusk was
artificial, in that clocks said it was still daytime—and
yet it was all too real.*

At the shore, the ocean turned silvery-black, reflecting the sky above.

Later came a rain of ashes. The fallout wiped away nothing, only making things blacker.

Soon the alarms faded and hordes of vampires emerged from their cellars . . . to claim their new world.

North River Tunnel

FET FOUND NORA sitting on the tracks in the bowels of the tunnel beneath the Hudson River. Nora's mother's head was in her lap, Nora stroking her gray hair while the sick woman slept.

"Nora," said Fet, sitting next to her, "come—let me help you, and your mother . . ."

"Mariela," said Nora. "Her name is Mariela." And then she broke down finally, crying, her body shuddering with deep, primal sobs as she buried her face in Fet's shoulder.

Eph soon returned from the eastbound tube, where he had been looking for Zack. Nora turned to him, spent, empty, almost rising but for her sleeping mother, hope and pain expressed on her face.

Eph pulled off the night-vision monocular and shook his head. Nothing.

Fet felt the tension between Eph and Nora. Each of them emotionally ravaged, and beyond words. Fet knew that Eph did not blame Nora, that there was no doubt Nora had done everything she could for Zack under the circumstances. But he also sensed that, in losing Zack, Nora had lost Eph too.

Fet retold the events leading up to Setrakian leaving with Gus for Locust Valley. "He told me to stay behind—to come here." Fet looked at Eph. "To find you."

Eph pulled a glass flask from his pocket, one he had found in the wheelhouse aboard the tugboat. He took a hard hit from it, then looked around the tunnel with an expression of angry disgust. "So here we are," he said.

Fet felt Nora bristle next to him. Then a distant roar began filling the tunnel. Fet couldn't track it at first, the sound distorted by the unceasing tone in his bad ear.

An engine, a motor, coming toward them—the noise a rumble of terror inside the long, stone tube.

Light approached. A train was impossible—wasn't it?

Two lights. Headlights. An automobile.

Fet pulled his sword, ready for anything. The big vehicle came to a stop, its thick tires shredded from the tracks, the black Hummer rattling along on its rims.

The front grill was white with vamp blood.

Gus climbed out. A blue bandanna was tied around his head. Fet hurried to the opposite door, looking for a passenger.

The Hummer was otherwise empty.

Gus saw whom Fet was looking for and shook his head.

"Tell me," said Fet.

Gus did. He told about leaving Setrakian at the nuclear power plant.

"You left him?" said Fet.

Gus's smile showed a flash of anger. "He demanded it. Same as he did of you."

Fet caught himself. He saw that the kid was right.

"He's gone?" said Nora.

"I don't see any other way," said Gus. "He was prepared to fight to the end. Angel stayed, that crazy fucker. No way the Master got away from those two without feeling some pain. If only radiation."

"Meltdown," said Nora.

Gus nodded. "I heard the blast and the sirens. Bad cloud headed this way. The old man said to get down here to you."

Fet said, "He sent us all here. To protect us from the fallout."

Fet looked around. Burrowed underground. He was used to having the upper hand in this scenario: the exterminator, gassing vermin in their holes. He looked around, thinking about what rats, the ultimate survivors, would do when faced with this situation—and he saw the derailed train in the distance, its bloodstained windows reflecting Gus's headlights.

"We'll clear out the train cars," he said. "We can sleep in there, in shifts, lock the doors. There's a café car we can raid for now. Water. Toilets."

"For a few days, maybe," said Nora.

"For as long as we can make it last," said Fet. He felt a surge of emotion—pride, resolve, gratitude, grief—striking him like a fist. The old man was gone; the old man lived on. "Long enough to let the worst of the radioactivity disperse up top."

"And then what?" Nora was beyond burned-out. She was done with this. With all of this. And yet there was no ending. Nowhere else to go, but on, and on, into this new hell on earth. "Setrakian is gone—dead, or possibly worse. There's a holocaust above us. They've won. The *strigoi* have prevailed. It's over. All over."

No one said anything. The air in the long tunnel hung still and silent.

Fet pulled his bag down off his shoulder. He opened it and rummaged through with dirty hands, then pulled out the silver-bound book.

"Maybe," he said. "Or—maybe not."

Eph grabbed one of Gus's strong flashlights and went off on his own again, following every trail of vampire waste to its end.

None of them brought him to Zack. Still, he went on, calling out his son's name, his voice echoing emptily through the tunnel, returning back to him like a taunt. He emptied the flask, and then hurled the thick glass at the tunnel wall, where the sound of its shattering was like a profanity.

Then he found Zack's inhaler.

Lying beside the track in an otherwise unremarkable stretch of tunnel. The prescription sticker was still affixed: *Zachary Goodweather, Kelton Street, Woodside, New York.* Suddenly, every one of those words spoke to him of things lost: name, street, neighborhood.

They had lost it all. These things meant nothing anymore.

Eph gripped the inhaler as he stood in the dark burrow beneath the earth. Gripped it so hard that the plastic casing started to crack.

He stopped then. *Preserve this,* he thought. He held it to his heart and switched off his flashlight. He stood still, vibrating with rage in the pure dark.

The world had lost the sun. Eph had lost his son.

Eph began to prepare himself for the worst.

He would return to the others. He would clear out the derailed train, and watch with them, and wait.

But while the others waited for the air to clear above, Eph would be waiting for something else.

He would be waiting for his Zack to return to him as a vampire.

He had learned from his mistake. He could not show any forbearance, as he had with Kelly.

It would be a privilege and a gift to release his only son.

But the worst thing that Eph had imagined—Zack's return as a vampire seeking his father's soul—turned out not to be the worst thing at all.

No.

The worst thing was—Zack never came.

The worst thing was the gradual realization that Eph's vigilance would have no end. That his pain would find no release.

The Night Eternal had begun.

The authors wish to acknowledge the assistance of Dr. Ilona Zsolnay of the Babylonian Section in the University Museum at the University of Pennsylvania.